In Sickness and In Health captured the highs and lows of the trials of cancer. This unique story had me laughing and crying. This book gives hope to those facing cancer or any other challenges or obstacles in their lives. I loved watching Luke and Michelle's faith grow stronger throughout the book. With each trial they faced, I could feel the raw emotions and pain and gained hope and peace right along with them. This book is an inspirational story that will leave you hopeful about the future!

-Rita Davenport,
Author, CSP, CPAE Award Winning Speaker, Entrepreneur

Both heart-breaking and heart-warming at the same time, this book is an excellent reminder that God provides enormous strength in times of struggle. Michelle Bader presents a difficult subject with, at times, laugh-out-loud humor that kept me wanting to turn the page into the next chapter of this inspiring couple's not-so-classic romance story. It is a "should read" for anyone in a committed relationship or anyone who wants to know what one looks like—and a "must read" for anyone facing life-altering health issues for themselves or someone they love.

-Kelly Soud Corsmeier,
retired Attorney and avid reader

Your writing is excellent. It has moved me very deeply. I just lost my wife to breast cancer six months ago, and reading what you wrote, I felt like I could directly relate to your feelings and experiences just as I went through something similar to you and felt and thought some of those same things as you did as I went through dealing with my wife's cancer and chemotherapy treatments. I hope that maybe someday, although I am not as good of a writer as you are, that maybe someday I will be able to find the strength to share my story as well. Reading your story has been both extremely wonderful and extremely painful at the same time, but I felt like I needed to read what you had written to help me deal with the loss of my wife and how amazing she was in dealing with her chemotherapy and fighting cancer and always staying so strong and positive through it all.

-Micheal Lyon,
English teacher, Okinawa, Japan

In Sickness and in Health

A Newlywed's Journey
Through *Faith*, *Love*, and *Cancer*

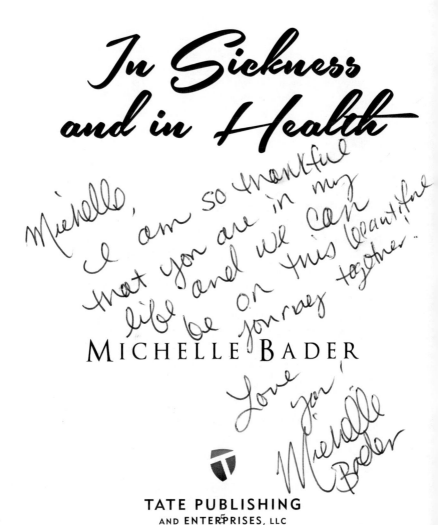

In Sickness and in Health

MICHELLE BADER

Michelle, I am so thankful that you are in my life and we can be on this beautiful journey together.

Love, you, Michelle Bader

TATE PUBLISHING
AND ENTERPRISES, LLC

Published by Tate Publishing & Enterprises, LLC
127 E. Trade Center Terrace | Mustang, Oklahoma 73064 USA
1.888.361.9473 | www.tatepublishing.com

Tate Publishing is committed to excellence in the publishing industry. The company reflects the philosophy established by the founders, based on Psalm 68:11,
"The Lord gave the word and great was the company of those who published it."

Book design copyright © 2013 by Tate Publishing, LLC. All rights reserved.
Cover design by Rodrigo Adolfo
Interior design by Jake Muelle

Published in the United States of America

ISBN: 978-1-62854-169-4
1. Biography & Autobiography / Personal Memoirs
2. Family & Relationships / Marriage
13.09.20

Dedication

*T*o my husband, Luke, and our three beautiful children: Hayden, Hayley, and Payton. I love you all so much and am thankful every day for you.

Also to my parents, Steve and Karen Rommel, you have always encouraged me in the process of writing this book and held my hand through every second of this journey. I couldn't have done it without you. I love you!

Table of Contents

A Princess in Pain

I couldn't breathe. I couldn't speak, I couldn't comprehend the depth of the words that were spoken to me. Cancer. *Cancer can't be happening to my family—my husband,* I thought desperately. *Not now, with a baby on the way and Luke and I only five months into our beautiful storybook marriage. Not possible!*

I closed my weary eyes and let myself bask in the memory of the past. I wanted to remember how it felt to be young and in love. I deeply wanted to go back to the favorite day I had ever experienced and be alive in that memory and as far away from the thought of cancer as I could.

The day I had been dreaming of for as long as I could remember had finally arrived. I stared in the mirror and admired the beauty of my wedding dress. I gazed at myself from every angle and watched the way my flowing gown swished as I moved. I adjusted my tiara and veil, and for the first time in my life, I truly felt like a princess. Butterflies stirred in my stomach as I thought of the most exciting part of being a princess— living happily ever after with my prince.

I looked down from the window I was standing next to. I could see the picturesque garden that I would be getting married in. Flowers bloomed in all directions and thousands of white lights were attached to the trees just waiting for nightfall to show their magical glow. My eyes followed the long pathway that led to the gazebo where Luke and I would be exchanging our vows. The gazebo was very large, large enough to fit two hundred of our guests. At the front of the gazebo I could just make out the top of the flower-filled arbor I would soon be standing under to become Mrs. Michelle Bader.

"Are you ready?" my mom asked me. "Luke is waiting."

My heart began to pound faster and faster as I anticipated seeing my soon-to-be husband.

"Yes. Will you help me with my dress?" I said as I pointed to the long, white, satin part of my dress that was lying on the floor. Mom quickly gathered it up and held it as we walked down the stairs. With each step I took, I felt as though I was floating higher and higher.

I walked to the doorway of the Victorian mansion that I had been getting ready in. I knew that Luke would be outside, anticipating me, his bride.

"Here I go." I opened the door and began my walk toward Luke.

Luke and I were having pictures before the wedding, so we had arranged to see each other privately. I could see Luke looking off into the distance as I walked toward him.

"Luke," I whispered softly.

Luke turned around and stared at me wide-eyed.

"You look so beautiful," he said softly, tenderly taking my hand in his own.

"You look very handsome yourself." I leaned up to kiss his cheek. We continued to stare at each other, and time seemed to stand still as our photographer began snapping pictures of us from all directions.

"Just pretend I'm not here," he said.

"Luke, look at the windows," I said as I pointed to the house. Through the window, I could see several faces gazing at us, trying to get a glimpse into our world. Luke looked over and laughed.

I love how he looks when he laughs, as though his eyes are dancing, I thought to myself.

We were soon joined by our eight bridesmaids, seven groomsmen, two candle lighters, two ring bearers, and one flower girl. The photographer took many pictures, and before I knew it, it was time to start the ceremony.

I watched from the beginning of the walkway as my wedding party made their way to the front of the gazebo. Soon the sounds of the "Wedding March" filled the air, and I knew my time had come to walk down the aisle.

"Are you ready, Dad?" I said as I linked my arm with his.

"Yes," he replied, and we began to walk slowly in time with the music.

My eyes locked on Luke, and he was all that I could see. *This is better than I ever dreamed it would be,* I thought as I floated toward my soon-to-be husband.

"Who gives this woman to this man?" the pastor asked when I reached the front of the gazebo.

"Her mother and I do, with our blessing," my dad said as he unlinked my arm from his, and I walked toward Luke. As I stood beside Luke, he took my hand in his. I looked at him and smiled, knowing this was the day I had waited for all of my life.

The pastor prayed a prayer of blessing over us, after which the sounds of one of my favorite songs "I Stand in Awe of You" flowed through the air. I lifted my hands to Jesus and felt more awe to the one I gave my heart to so many years ago than I ever had before. I felt awe that God had set aside Luke to be my husband. I felt awe because God had given me more of a prince than I had ever dreamed of. I was in awe of the way God had carefully orchestrated this union—the most sacred union of all—husband and wife.

When it was time to say our vows, I faced Luke.

"I, Michelle, take you, Luke, to be my husband from this moment on." *Husband.* I liked the way that sounded.

"In hardships and in triumphs," my voice strained to say the words. Tears were freely flowing.

"In poverty or in wealth." I continued to cry.

"In sickness and in health." I said the words without even the slightest clue of the sickness we were soon to endure.

"I vow to love you and to care for you all the days of my life." I meant each and every word of those vows with all of my heart.

Luke repeated the same vows to me through teary eyes.

"Luke and Michelle wish to participate in two very special acts to express their love and devotion to

God and to each other. The unity candle expresses God's work in making the two one flesh. Also, they want their first act to be one of communion with their LORD, establishing their married relationship on their relationship with Jesus," the pastor explained to our near three hundred guests.

As the song "My Jesus, I love Thee" began to play, Luke and I each took a candle in our hands and together lit our unity candle. As the music continued, the pastor led us through communion.

"This is Jesus's body broken for you," he said as we took a piece of bread and remembered what Jesus had done for us by bringing us to this day.

"This is Jesus's blood poured out for you. Drink in remembrance of him," he said as we drank our tiny cups of grape juice.

Luke took my hand and whispered in my ear, "I want to pray with you."

"Jesus, thank you for this day that we could be joined together," he spoke into my ear while the music played. "Please help our love to always be honoring to you. I know that you have been with us every step of the way and will continue to be throughout our marriage, no matter what hardships we may encounter. Please bless this marriage. We love you. Amen." I looked up to see him wipe away a tear from his cheek.

The music ended and the pastor began to speak.

"Ladies and gentleman, I am honored to be the first to present to you Mr. and Mrs. Luke Bader."

Our friends and family began to clap.

"Luke, you may kiss your bride."

Luke leaned down and kissed me gently and softly.

The ceremony was complete. Luke grabbed my hand and we walked down the aisle. It was official. We were married. We were soon overwhelmed with talking to hundreds of guests, and the night wore on quickly. I looked up in the trees and saw the magical glow of thousands of tiny white lights. The gazebo was now lit up as well, and I felt as though I was in a magical wonderland. As we greeted our guests, the chairs from the gazebo were removed, and it was turned into a dance floor.

"If I could please have your attention," I heard a faraway voice on a microphone say. "Please join us as Michelle and Luke have their first dance as husband and wife."

Luke and I quickly walked back to the gazebo. As we were in the middle, our song began. I wrapped my arms around Luke's neck as he put his around my waist. We danced, oblivious to the eyes that watched our every move. As the music played, I thought about the words as I sang them to Luke.

The song said exactly what I was feeling—that Luke was my once in a lifetime chance.

As I sang, Luke danced freely and with more life than I had ever seen before. He spun me around and pulled me close in his arms again. *I want to remember and cherish this moment forever,* I thought to myself as the music faded to a stop.

The night continued as we cut the cake, danced with family and friends, and threw the garter and bouquet. Soon it was time to leave. Luke and I walked hand in hand to our getaway car. Hundreds of tiny bubbles flew at us in the air as we departed. It was truly the princess day that I dreamed of my entire life.

"Baby, baby, are you okay?" Luke said to me, and I was quickly brought back to the present—the present that now included cancer. My tears began to fall as I reached out to Luke. I lay my head on his chest and listened to the sound of his heartbeat. "Please God, help us. Help us survive this. Help me. I don't think I can do this." I cried out to God, and I knew he was listening. He had never left me my entire life, and I knew this time would be no different. Cancer was not something that I thought would become part of my everyday thoughts, and it did not yet seem like a reality. *God, what else have you planned for us?* I asked silently. The soft words I had heard so many times flowed into my head at that moment.

"For I know the plans I have for you declares the Lord, plans to prosper you and not to harm you , plans to give you a hope and a future" (Jeremiah 29:11, NIV).

The words gave me peace for the future and calmed me for the present. "Thank you Jesus, thank you for your plans," I prayed. I opened my eyes and prepared to face the future, no matter what it may bring.

Shock

My princess day was over, but my fairy tale had just begun. Luke and I went to Maui for ten days for our honeymoon. We took long walks on the beach and enjoyed romantic sunsets followed by evenings of love and laughter. We went scuba diving and held hands as we watched the wonders of the sea. The luau that we attended had a spectacular view, and the waterfalls we swam under were amazing. It was a trip to paradise.

While on the honeymoon, I received a call from one of the schools where I was interviewed before the wedding. I was offered a job to teach kindergarten. This was another blessing from God. I had been through seven interviews that summer and was ready to settle down with a job. When I returned home, I was instantly involved in a whirlwind of activities preparing to teach.

It was exciting being newlyweds and living in our new house together. I found myself calling Luke "husband" many times. I loved telling people I was married and enjoyed hearing my students call me "Mrs." Being a wife was everything I had ever dreamed of. There was no better feeling than knowing that I would be waking up to Luke every day.

That fall was a busy and eventful time. Fall has always been Luke's favorite season. He loved the feel of the cool, crisp air and the sound and sights of football games. For several years, Luke had enjoyed watching his favorite football team, the Oregon Ducks, play. He would always make a day of it, sometimes leaving at a crazy time like 3:00 a.m. to see them play. This season was no different. I even tried to go with him one time, but after one quarter I knew that I never wanted to go again. Watching football was not something that I enjoyed!

One Saturday night, Luke was watching the Ducks play, and I walked in from an evening out where I had found out that a friend was pregnant, and I decided that I wanted to take a pregnancy test. I guess it was a pretty important part of the game, but Luke followed me into the bathroom anyway. I stared very hard at the test trying to decide if I was seeing one pink line or two. "Luke, Luke, do you think it is two?" I asked him excitedly. Luke said he wasn't sure but that when the game was over, we could go get another test. Finally, the game ended, and we went out and bought another pregnancy test. We got home, took the test and knew for sure: We were going to be parents! It was not what we had planned, but God had different plans for us.

At that time, Luke was working at a local post office. God had placed him there for a specific reason. He had many coworkers who had been praying for him and encouraging him for years. He had several mentors and friends who had helped him to grow closer to God. Luke had a new mail route, which involved nine miles of walking. He would come home exhausted. He continued on this route for several months. As the days and months went by, he noticed a swelling and sharp pain in his right ankle. He would come home and put an ice pack on it, but the pain persisted every day. One December day, Luke decided it was time to go to the doctor to get his ankle examined.

As Luke waited in the exam room, he could hear the doctors whispering to each other as they looked at his x-ray.

"That is bad. How old is he?" one doctor said.

"Just twenty-five," the other doctor replied. Luke knew from the sound of things that something was very wrong. He came home and kept to himself how bad he really thought it was. He was sent to a specialist for further examination. The specialist agreed that something was wrong and wanted Luke to have a biopsy.

The day of the biopsy arrived. At this point, I was still very optimistic. I thought it was going to be something that would be an easy fix. I had no idea what it was but convinced myself that everything would be fine. Luke and I went to the preop room and waited for further instructions. A nurse came in and asked him when the last time he ate was.

He replied with, "This morning."

"What?" she said. "You were supposed to not eat for twelve hours!" This was not clearly communicated to us, and because of that, we had to wait another five hours before the surgery could begin.

Luke's biopsy finally began. Hours went by, and then I was able to see him. He was in a lot of pain where they had opened up his ankle to do the biopsy. The car ride home was bumpy, and Luke cringed in pain

Michelle Bader

at every bump. When we got home, we had a pleasant surprise. We had ordered a baby heart monitor to listen to our baby's heartbeat. It was waiting for us on our front doorstep.

I will never forget the look on Luke's face the first time he heard the sound of our baby's heart. His eyes grew wide, and he was amazed. There was truly a little miracle growing inside of me.

The days after the biopsy were the beginning of many painful days to come. Luke has always had a hard time asking for help. Being on crutches and depending on me to help him was a struggle for him. Each day we anticipated a call from Luke's surgeon to tell us the result of the biopsy. Finally, two weeks later, we received a call from her. I answered the phone. She asked for us both to be on the phone, and my heart began to beat faster. Luke and I both sat on our bed holding hands and listening on two different phones.

"Hi, guys. Well, we found out from the biopsy that this is a very rare form of bone cancer, so rare in fact that we have sent it to New York to examine it further. I know this is difficult to hear."

Did she just say cancer? My head was spinning, this could *not* be happening! Many big words were flying around—*oncologist, tumor, mesenchymal chondrosarcoma, Ewing's*—my mind could not keep up. I felt like I was paralyzed, in a nightmare. I tried to wake myself up. *Wake up, Michelle,* I told myself, *This isn't real, just wake up!* As hard as I tried, I could not wake up. I looked at my husband as we continued to listen to the doctor speak of things that were new and foreign to us. We hung up the phone. We wrapped our arms around each other and cried. My heart had never known such pain. I was more scared than I had ever been in my life.

Cancer. The word was so scary. Cancer takes people's lives. Cancer destroys. I hated cancer. I felt angry—angry that we were going to have to battle one of the most devastating diseases in the world. Why did this have to happen to my sweet husband? Of all the people in the world, why him?

I felt numb. I was in complete shock. I felt anger seeping into every part of me. The tears continued to flow as my world fell apart. That night was a sleepless, restless night. The next day, we had an appointment with an oncologist. At that point, I didn't even know what an oncologist was. I came to find out that an oncologist specializes in the treatment of cancer.

Luke's mom picked us up for the appointment. My heart was bleeding inside as we drove. I entered the medical office as if I were on autopilot. My heart beat faster as I walked up the stairs to the office. In the office, there was a feeble-looking woman with a scarf on her head. Sitting across from her was a sad, frail man who looked too weak to stand. I dropped my head and silently cried out to God, *Where are you? Why did you let this happen to my husband? I am so angry!*

We sat in silence as we waited for Luke's name to be called. We were finally called back to a cold, empty office where we were soon greeted by the oncologist. He began to speak of Luke's cancer called mesenchymal chondrosarcoma. He explained that it was a very rare bone cancer most often found in children. It was so rare, in fact, that they did not know how to treat it. I did not find these words comforting. He went on to tell us they wanted to treat Luke with very aggressive chemotherapy. *Chemotherapy* had always been a word that made me cringe. I didn't know much about it, but I knew I never wanted it to be a part of my daily vocabulary.

I fought to hold back tears as he divulged the details of the complications of chemotherapy. Hair loss was to be the least of the side effects. He began to talk of the dangers of having a fever or even an everyday cold. My tears began to flow as he said there was a risk of not being able to have more children. Images of our future children began to crumble. I felt overwhelmed and scared. He continued to tell us that he would like Luke to do a full year of treatment. I could not believe my ears! How could Luke be treated for a full year? That was way too long. The oncologist told us that they would begin treatment after they took a few blood tests and did a CAT scan. The first treatment was to be a one-day outpatient and the next was to be a five-day hospital stay.

The appointment finally ended. I felt sick and ready to collapse at any moment. We returned home, and I tried to let the reality of the situation sink in. Yes, my husband had cancer and I was going to have to be strong and help him get through it. I was so used to Luke being the strong one that this was going to be a new and difficult job for me.

Every day, my anger grew a little more. Each time a person would ask me about Luke, I would get a little angrier. I felt that the people asking me about him were saying it as a courtesy to me rather than because they really cared. I would go to work and look at everyone around me and see that their lives were going so well, and I would get angry. I would pick people out of a crowd and think to myself, *Why not that person? Why doesn't he have cancer? Why not that ungrateful person who has never done a bit of good in his whole life? Why not them? Why my husband, the most wonderful person in the world?*

I was nervous the day that Luke went to have his CAT scan done. There is always the fear that the cancer may be somewhere else too. Luke fit his body into a very tiny machine that looked inside of him. When he was done, the CAT scan specialist told him to go wash his forehead because it looked like there might be something there. He later told me that he was very frightened that there were cancer cells in his brain. They checked again and found that what was showing up on the CAT scan was from a sinus infection. What a relief that was!

Learning to deal with cancer in our lives was a challenge. Luke prepared to begin chemotherapy. I was nervous about what would happen to Luke during chemo and how I would cope with him being sick. The day of the first chemo treatment arrived. It was to be an outpatient treatment, so Luke didn't think it was necessary for me to miss work to be there. He sat on a chair and had an IV put in his vein. For five hours, he was pumped with poison intended to kill the cancer cells in his body. Along with killing bad cells, it also kills good ones. Hour after hour, he watched the fluid drip into his veins and felt a burning sensation as it permeated through his arm and body.

I came home to him that night, and he was acting surprisingly well. There was no sign of nausea. I was very happy that he was doing well and ready to continue fighting the battle against cancer. But there was still a very long way to go and many more chemotherapy treatments to undergo. We decided to take things one day at a time and not be overwhelmed by the unknown.

Our Child

A few weeks after Luke's first chemo treatment, we had an appointment to have an ultrasound of our baby. I could feel my heart beating faster and faster with anticipation to see my baby for the first time. As my mom and I waited in the waiting room for my name to be called, I looked at my watch again. Where was Luke? He was coming straight from a doctor's appointment where he was getting a second opinion about everything.

When Luke arrived, he looked tired again; I could see it in his eyes. "I had to rush to make it here," he said. As he entered the office, I heard my name being called.

"Here we go, baby!" I said excitedly to Luke.

Luke and I were ushered into a small room, and I was instructed to dress in a hospital-style gown. I quickly changed and lay on the table. I looked around the dimly lit room and viewed a screen which I assumed would be where I would see my baby.

"Knock, knock," I heard a woman's voice say. "Are you ready?"

I lay on the bed as my gown was lifted, and I felt a cold gooey liquid being applied to my stomach. With a flick of a switch, the screen turned on. Suddenly, I was able to see my baby! Tears welled up in my eyes.

Luke squeezed my hand and said, "Oh, wow!"

I gazed into Luke's deep-brown eyes and said, "That's our baby!"

For a moment, all the things that lay heavily on my heart seemed far away. All I could see was the miracle growing inside of me. I was filled with awe and wonder as I watched my baby move around.

My thoughts were suddenly interrupted by the question we had been waiting for. "Do you want to know the sex?"

"Yes," we replied in unison.

"You are having a boy."

Luke looked at me, and I knew he was overjoyed.

"Hayden," I whispered. "Hayden Luke Bader."

We continued to look at our baby boy. Many pictures were taken and the doctor explained what all the images were. Then the viewing of Hayden was over too quickly and it was time to go.

My mom was still in the waiting room waiting to hear the news.

"It's a boy," I said quickly.

She squealed in delight and hugged me tightly. She handed me a gift bag with little blue shoes and a tiny blue frame.

"How did you know?" I asked, amazed.

"I didn't," she replied. She lifted up another pink gift bag with pink items inside. We looked at each other and laughed.

That day was the first day in a long time that I truly felt joy; the first time I was able to take my mind off cancer and the unknown and focus on my baby—my beautiful baby boy. He was the most beautiful thing I had ever laid eyes on, and I had the ultrasound pictures to prove it. I put the pictures in a small green album with rattles on it and carried it everywhere with me. I began showing these pictures to anyone and everyone I met.

February continued, and each day I grew more excited about our baby boy. Luke would often lay his head on my stomach and talk to Hayden. "How's my baby boy?" Luke would say excitedly. Hayden was our one escape from the reality of cancer.

Valentine's Day was approaching. Luke was scheduled to have a round of chemo the day before, so I was counting on not being able to go out for dinner. To my surprise, Luke was feeling better than he expected and we were able to go to one of my favorite Italian restaurants, Little Italy.

The lights in the restaurant were dim as we were led to our booth. I looked around and noticed that there was only one other couple in the restaurant. As we sat down, visions of a similar restaurant filled my mind…

The sound of the ocean set the mood for one of our first meals as husband and wife. The breeze played with my hair, and my heart felt as light as the wind. I stared across the table at my husband, *my* husband!

"Luke," I said slowly.

"Yes, baby," Luke replied.

"Things are going really well for us! I mean, we just got married; we have a beautiful house to go home to, a wonderful family, and today I was offered a full-time teaching position!" I excitedly said.

"I know, sweetie, we have a lot to be thankful for."

"We are so lucky!"

"Not lucky, baby, blessed," Luke corrected me.

"Blessed," I said as I watched another wave crash against the sandy shore. I observed the sun paint the sky colors so vibrant that they could come only from the hand of God, the creator of all blessings.

"Baby, you know how the Bible talks about going through seasons of life? Well, I believe this is our good season. If and when things ever get difficult for us, we need to remember this. We need to remember the joy we are experiencing now," I said.

My loving husband gazed into my eyes and said, "You are right, baby!"

My thoughts were interrupted by the waitress asking me what I wanted to order. As Luke looked over the menu, I studied him with my eyes. How faraway that day in Maui felt now. How faraway did our good season seem. I looked at my husband and felt a sadness sweep across my body. I noticed that his hair was beginning to fall out. There were pieces of it missing. I was not sad because of the hair loss but sad because it made him look like he was sick. His eyes also looked tired, and his skin was a paler complexion than normal. Looking at him once again confirmed what I already knew to be true: We were, in fact, in the hard season of life, and it had only just begun.

Hotel Sunnyside

❧❧❧

"Hey, baby, are you ready to join me at Hotel Sunnyside?" Luke said to me over the phone in a joking voice.

"Yes, how is it?" I replied as I gathered the last of my things into my overnight bag. Had I remembered everything? I had a nervous, anxious feeling in the pit of my stomach. I laughed to myself at the fact that Luke was referring to Sunnyside Hospital as "Hotel Sunnyside." Despite everything going on, Luke was still able to keep a positive attitude about everything. He was such a good example to me.

"Well, we ended up getting a private room, and there is a bed for you."

"Good," I said as I shut the door of my yellow bug. "I will be there soon, baby. I love you."

"I love you too."

I began the short journey to the hospital. I had wanted to go with Luke in the morning when he had gone, but he insisted he would be okay and that I should go to work. It had been difficult to concentrate at work that day knowing my husband was in the hospital having his first inpatient chemo treatment. I never told my students what was going on with Luke, but a few of the parents knew, and they were very supportive. When the students asked why I was gone so many days, I simply told them that my husband was sick and I needed to stay with him. I continued driving as I mentally prepared myself to see for the first time my husband receiving a chemo treatment.

I arrived in the hospital within twenty minutes and parked my car in the hospital's parking garage. I brought along as many things as my arms could hold—things we might need during the hospital stay. I entered the hospital and immediately found a sign saying Oncology Department. I took a right turn and began my journey down a long empty hallway. I had to stop halfway down the hall and readjust all of my things. As I looked down at my overstuffed bag, pillow, blanket, and body pillow, I realized that maybe I over packed. But we were staying for five days. I was starting to get uncomfortable sleeping at night with my growing baby taking up so much room, so I had to have a body pillow to make the sleeping easier.

I picked my things back up and continued down the hall. I came upon two large doors which appeared to be locked. I looked around for someone to help me. I found a nurse, and she told me to go ahead through the doors. As I opened the door to the chemotherapy wing, my stomach was in knots. Nurses were busy walking back and forth and checking charts. I walked past the first room and continued on. The next door on the left said "Bader." There was also a shocking neon-orange sign which said "Warning: Chemotherapy in Progress" and another that said "Please wash your hands when entering the room." These signs made me feel even more uneasy.

Slowly and cautiously, I reached for the cold silver door handle and opened the door. My husband looked up from a newspaper he was reading and said, "Hey, baby."

"Hi," I replied as I leaned over to kiss him.

I studied my husband. He was lying on a hospital bed that was propped up so he was in the sitting position. Attached to his right arm just above his wrist, on the underside, was a thin tube. The tube was hooked to him through a needle in his vein. I have always been a person who feels faint even at the thought of a needle. I was surprised when I didn't feel dizzy looking at his arm. I could hear the *swish, pump, swish, pump* sound of the chemotherapy drugs being pumped into Luke. I followed the tubes up with my eyes and saw that they were attached to a plastic-like bag which hung from a pole.

I found a chair to Luke's left and sat down. I was surprised to find that it reclined and was happy to be able to put my feet up and rest them for a while.

"So, this is Hotel Sunnyside, huh?" I said with an upbeat tone in my voice.

"Ya, it's not that bad. The chair you are sitting on folds into a bed," Luke replied.

I looked down and tried to see how the tiny chair that I was sitting in could turn into a bed and be comfortable for me and my growing baby. I looked at my husband and instantly felt ashamed of my thoughts. I knew he was more uncomfortable than me with a needle in his arm.

"This is one of the very few private rooms in the whole chemo ward. We told them that I had a pregnant wife coming to stay with me, and they gave it to me.

They did say that we may have to move if someone who is sicker than me checks in and needs a private room. There are some people who have such a low immune system from all the chemo drugs that they cannot be in a room with anyone else," Luke said.

"I am glad we got this room. I wouldn't like to share with anyone else," I replied. I knew how much Luke valued his privacy, and having a private room was important to him.

Our conversation was interrupted when a woman in scrubs entered the room.

"Hi," she said. "You must be Luke's wife, I am Christy, Luke's nurse for the next four hours.

"Hi, I am Michelle."

"I understand you will be staying here tonight."

"Yes, all of the nights," I replied.

"Let me know if you need anything. Oh, and please don't use the bathroom."

Luke and I looked at each other. I knew we were thinking the same thing, that that request would be near impossible.

"Really?" I asked. "Even during the night? I am pregnant and that would be really hard to do."

"Well, just a minute. I will go ask the head nurse," she said quickly and left the room only to return a few minutes later. "I spoke with our head nurse, and she said to use the other bathroom down the hall and out the doors when you can, but at night you can use the bathroom in the room as long as you flush it first."

"Okay, just curious, but why do I need to flush it first?"

"To make sure that all remains of the drugs that are in Luke's urine are flushed away and have no way of being in contact with you," she said.

"Well, thank you. I will remember to flush first!" I said with a smile. She left the room, and Luke and I looked at each other and laughed. This cancer thing was turning out to be quite an adventure.

Throughout the evening, we had many visitors come to see us, including Luke's and my parents. When everyone left, we cuddled together on his little hospital bed and watched a movie. It wasn't very comfortable, but we were together and that was what mattered.

Nurses continue to come in and out of the room and check how Luke was doing. When Luke's chemo drugs ran out, we would hear an annoying *beep*, *beep* from the machine signaling that it was time to call the nurse. Two nurses would come in and get another bag of chemotherapy medicine. They would check the label on the drugs to see if it matched the hospital band that he was wearing on his wrist.

The chemo continued for close to fourteen hours. My ears quickly became accustomed to the *swish*, *pump*, *swish*, *pump* of the machine, and I could no longer distinguish it from other sounds in the room.

Around midnight, I fell asleep on my little reclining chair that turned into a bed. I woke up a few times during the night and had to remind myself where I was. I, of course, had to use the bathroom and stumbled around Luke's bed to find the bathroom in the dark. The floor felt cold on my feet and the room smelled a distinct smell that only a hospital can have. I fell back asleep quickly and dreamed of happier days.

I woke up as the sun shone on my face. I looked over at my husband and smiled. He was already awake.

"Happy birthday, baby," Luke said with a smile.

That's right, it was my birthday. The hospital was not where I thought I would be spending my twenty-fifth birthday.

Birthdays have always been a big deal in my family. My mom had always gone out of her way to make sure that my birthdays were special and memorable. This year had been no different. My mind drifted to the events of a week ago.

"Are you ready for dinner, baby?" Luke said to me.

"Yes, I am coming," I replied.

We were going out to eat with my parents at a new restaurant in town called Ruby Tuesdays. We drove less than a mile to the restaurant. Upon reaching the place, we were ushered straight to the back into a large room. I opened the doors.

"Surprise!"

My mouth dropped open in shock as I saw before me many of my family and friends. I looked around the room and saw about twenty-five people. My mom had thrown surprise parties for me before, and I usually had some clue that they were coming. This time I was really taken by surprise.

I began to greet and talk to all the guests. I looked over at Luke and noticed how tired and sick he looked. It saddened my heart to see him that way. The party continued and I was given many wonderful gifts, ate cake, and was embarrassed by a game of "Michelle trivia" that my family had made up. It was a great distraction from the upcoming chemo treatment, where I would be on my birthday. I was once again thankful for my wonderful family who always went above and beyond what I ever expected.

Here I was, on my birthday, in the hospital. I watched as a nurse took Luke's breakfast order. She was very surprised at the amount of food that he ordered. Apparently most chemo patients do not have the kind of appetite that Luke had.

"Would you like anything?" the nurse said to me.

"No, thank you." I strained to see her. All I could see was a blur where I knew her face should be. I did not have my contacts on and could not make out even simple objects that were close to me.

The nurse soon returned with Luke's breakfast. He was very happy to eat it. He doused everything in ketchup and enjoyed his meal. I decided that I was not going to be able to go back to sleep, so I got dressed and put my contacts in. I walked to the front of the hospital and bought a newspaper for Luke. When I returned, I found that he already had one that a nurse had given him. The morning wore on, and my mom came to take me out to lunch and go shopping. She had always taken me shopping on my birthdays since I was seven. I kissed my husband good-bye and left him to continue his chemo.

"I will be back soon, baby. Call if you need anything," I said.

"Okay. I love you," Luke replied.

"I love you too," I said as I walked toward the door. I felt guilty leaving Luke to go shopping while he had a needle pumping poison into his body, but he said he would be fine and he wanted me to go.

My mom and I had a wonderful lunch and a good time shopping. I bought many maternity clothes as I was quickly outgrowing the clothes that I had. While we were shopping, there was an underlying tone of sadness.

"Next year, I hope my birthday will be better. Luke will not be on chemo, and Hayden will be eight months old. I pray it is," I said to my mom as we drove back to the hospital.

"I am sure it will be. You have a baby to look forward to," my mom replied. We pulled into the parking garage in the hospital.

I returned to Luke and immediately began showing him the new things I had purchased. With each outfit, he continued to nod and say that he liked it. In the midst of my showing him my things, a nurse came in and had to switch arms that he was receiving chemo in. He had a needle that stayed in his arm twenty-four hours a day, and after about a day and a half his vein would get tired, and they would have to switch it to a vein from the other arm.

My birthday in the hospital continued, and we ordered pizza for dinner. When the pizza arrived, the nurses made comments about it, and we shared it with some of them. We were starting to realize that we were different from the other chemo patients who stayed in the hospital. Several nurses had already commented to Luke that it was nice to see someone so positive for a change. Luke would always reply that his peace came from God.

My husband became a light to everyone around him. He inspired me to turn to God more and put away my anger. He showed me what it meant to look to God and be thankful in every situation.

My birthday was not one that I had expected, but I learned more on that birthday from husband than I ever had in my life.

The chemo continued for three more days, and we went home exhausted and prepared for the aftermath and side effects of the chemo that would soon show its face.

Chemo Effects

Luke and I returned home after five long days in the hospital. We tried to go back to our usual routine, but there was nothing usual about Luke suffering from the chemo effects. The first morning back at work after staying in the hospital, I felt as though I was caught in a fog. A thick haze seemed to cover everything I looked at.

I was amidst my twenty kindergarten students, trying to give them my all, when my mind wandered back to the events of the morning. I cringed as I thought of what I had seen Luke do as I was leaving.

Seated at the kitchen table was my wonderful husband getting ready to give himself a shot.

"Hey, baby," Luke said.

"Yes, baby," I replied.

"Would you get me the needles out of the refrigerator?"

"Sure." I opened the door of our white refrigerator and scanned the contents. On the top shelf, I found a brown paper bag that held the needles. I pulled one out; it was long and surprisingly thick. *How is he going to do this?* I thought to myself.

"Here you go, baby," I handed him the needle. "How many days do you have to do this?"

"Ten days, twice a day," Luke replied with an unmistakable sadness in his voice.

"Can I be alone to do this?" Luke said as he pulled up his pants and got ready to put the needle in his thigh.

"Yes, I am on my way out. I love you," I said, kissing him lightly.

"I love you too," Luke said as I walked out the door.

"Mrs. Bader, he hit me," a piercingly high voice screeched. I was instantly reminded of where I was as I heard the ever-so-popular kindergarten complaint. My mind returned to the present as I investigated the concern. Two and a half hours passed and I was relieved that I had made it to lunch. I couldn't wait to call Luke and see how he was doing.

I picked up the phone, remembering to dial nine to get out and waited to hear my husband's voice. *Ring, ring, ring.* After five rings, I finally hung up. *Well, I* thought, *he is probably asleep. I am glad he is able to rest.* I looked at the clock; I still had twenty minutes until my next class would show up.

I grabbed my lunch and headed to the staff room. I walked quickly hoping to avoid anyone asking me how Luke was doing. I made it without any encounters. I sat down quietly and tried to make myself invisible. My only purpose there was to eat my lunch as quick as possible and to return to my classroom unnoticed.

I listened to the conversation around me and thought how petty and unimportant the things being discussed were. *How can these people just go on with all of their lives, when my world has been devastated?* I silently screamed while smiling at those around me.

"How is your husband?" a coworker said to me from across the table.

I tried to think of what to say. Should I tell her the truth? Tell her about the agonizing nights in the hospital? Tell her how I was scared to death of what cancer could do to Luke, me, my baby?

"He is doing good under the circumstances," I replied. "He hasn't thrown up from the chemo yet, so that is a good thing," I said quickly, trying to cover any hint of emotion in my voice.

"That is good," she replied.

I promptly got up and threw away the remains of my lunch. I walked back to my classroom and for every person I saw, I would wonder if they knew what was going on in my life. I continued through the day and was ready to leave at exactly 3:30. I made the twenty-minute drive home and entered our house.

"Luke," I called out.

Silence. I walked through the hall to our bedroom. As I opened the door, I saw Luke sleeping on the bed. Sun streamed in through the window and landed on his pale face. I stood frozen, watching him breathe. His hair was now completely gone. After many mornings of waking up to find hair on his pillow and sheets, he had decided to shave it off. I had come home from work one day to find all of his hair gone. I cried as I looked at him and he held me. I explained to him that it was not that he didn't look good, but rather it was a tangible effect of chemo that was now visible to all. A warm tear made its way down my face as I continued to watch him. He still had a few eyelashes and just a hint of eyebrows. His once hairy chest was now bare.

Suddenly, I felt a movement from within. Hayden was kicking me. Once, twice, he continued moving and dancing within me. I placed my hand on my stomach. *Thank you, God, for giving me Hayden and reminding me that things will get better,* I silently prayed. Luke's eyes began to flutter open.

"Hey baby," I said excitedly. "Hayden is kicking. Do you want to feel?" I walked quickly over to the bed and placed his hand on my stomach.

"Wow," Luke said with wide eyes. He had only felt Hayden move a few times and was still amazed to feel him. I lay down beside Luke, and he put his head on my stomach and began to talk to our unborn miracle.

"How's my boy?" Luke said as he was kicked on the cheek by Hayden. We looked at each other and laughed. It seemed that Hayden liked hearing the sound of his daddy's voice. Luke continued talking to Hayden for several minutes, with Hayden responding each time with a kick. I knew then that God was already forming a bond between Luke and our precious baby boy.

"I tried to call you," I said to Luke when he was done talking to Hayden.

"I was probably asleep. I was so tired today I could barely get out of bed."

"How are you feeling now?"

"Still tired and a little nauseous."

"I am sorry. Do you want me to make you any dinner?" I asked.

"No, thank you. Nothing sounds good," replied Luke.

"I know the feeling," I said, thinking about my first trimester of pregnancy when I was so hungry but there was nothing that sounded good enough to eat.

Our days and evenings continued in pretty much the same way. The only thing that varied for Luke was that twice a week he would have to go to the doctor and get his blood samples taken. This was done in order to know what his blood counts were. If he had particularly low counts, then we knew not to go out anywhere.

As a kindergarten teacher, I was always worried about bringing home germs. I would always thoroughly wash my hands before going home. One day, as I was going about my normal routine at work of getting the kids lined up at the door, I heard a child say "Who are you?"

I turned around to see my wonderful husband at the door.

"I'm Mrs. Bader's husband," Luke replied.

I smiled at him and said hi. I continued getting the kids lined up. "I will be right back," I told Luke as I exited my classroom door.

As soon as the kids were all in their correct buses, I went back to my classroom excited at the thought of Luke being there.

"What are you doing here?" I entered the room and kissed my husband.

"I wanted to bring you lunch and tell you I love you," Luke said as he held up one of my favorite pregnancy foods—a cheeseburger from AM/PM.

"You are the best!" I hugged him tightly. Suddenly, I remembered that he was not supposed to be around germs.

"Baby, a school is not a good place for you to be in right now!" I said in a worried tone.

"I will be okay," Luke said.

We pulled up two small chairs and sat down at a child-sized table. I looked at Luke trying to sit comfortably in a chair made for a five-year-old and laughed.

"Sorry, baby. All we have here are little chairs!" I said.

We ate together for the next twenty minutes, and Luke said he needed to be going, and I told him that it would be a good idea for him to be gone before the next group of kids and germs arrived. I said good-bye to him and thought about what a wonderful husband he was. Most husbands do not even think about being so sweet as to bring their wives lunch at work, let alone coming to the school while on the effects of chemo. I was blessed, and I knew it. Despite all the things we were going through, I knew God had given me the best of the best. I was thankful once again for Luke's positive attitude and outlook on all the things going on in our life. He helped me keep things in perspective and often reminded me that things could always be worse.

While my husband appeared to be stable and strong in his outlook and attitude, I continued to be a storm of emotions. One day I could be happy and positive about everything, and the next day something could happen, and I would once again divulge in my anger and bitterness. Very few people really knew the extent of what was going on inside of me.

A few weeks passed and Luke was starting to feel better. It was almost time for Luke to have another round of chemo. I hated how he would start getting over the effects of chemo, and then right when he was feeling good, he would have to have another round.

This time, Luke received the one-day outpatient chemo to which he went alone. He liked getting the chemo over in one day as opposed to stretched over five days. He went to the oncologist, as scheduled, where his ever-faithful mom met him. His mom was always very good about taking Luke to appointments and thinking of everything that we needed help for.

That day was no different. His mom brought him lunch and also left him alone, as she knew he liked to have his space. As Luke watched his mother leave, he thought of what it must be like to be a parent of a son with cancer. Luke thought back to the ultrasound of Hayden and the times he had felt Hayden move and respond to his voice. For the first time in his life, he saw things from a parent's perspective. He realized what he had heard so many times was really true: You can't understand how deep your love can be until you are a parent.

Luke thought of what it would be like if Hayden was sick and how he would do anything in the world to take away that pain for him if he could. That day,

Luke had gained a whole new perspective on what it must be like for his parents to see him have cancer. He knew they would do anything to take it away, just as he would for Hayden.

Luke returned home and continued with his after-chemo routines. One day, he received a call from the doctor who had done the biopsy and discovered the cancer. She said that we had a decision to make. The cancer was in his ankle and needed to be removed one way or another. There were two options. The first was to do a surgery in which the cancer was cut out and new bone would be added where the cancer had eaten away at Luke's ankle. The second was to have a below-the-knee amputation. With the first option, Luke would have to be on crutches for at least a year and then wear a special boot for the rest of his life, and there would be a higher risk for the cancer returning. The second option, in my mind, was just plain unthinkable!

We were told that we had to make a decision within the next few weeks. How could we make that kind of life-changing decision in such a short span of time? We were overwhelmed and cried out to God for answers.

Decisions

❧❧❧

I looked around the waiting room in the doctor's office. It was not an appointment for Luke but to check how my pregnancy was going. In the beginning, I looked forward to these appointments; but as my weight climbed up the scale higher and higher, the focus of my appointment became more about my weight gain than about my pregnancy.

As I scanned the room and sized up the other women, I thought I looked like a bloated whale sitting next to them. I wondered if any of the women in the room were going through anything like me. I doubted that any pregnant woman knew what it was like to face what I was up against.

The familiar melody of my phone rang, and I quickly answered it before it would disturb anyone. I looked at the caller ID and was happy to see that it was Luke. I knew he has an appointment as well, and I was anxious to hear how it went.

"Hello," I said.

"Hi, baby," Luke said with a sad tone in his voice.

"How was your appointment?"

"Depressing. We went over my options; they don't sound very good. I will explain it more to you when you get home,"

"Okay," I replied, still overwhelmed by the life-altering decision we had to make.

"Michelle Bader," I heard a nurse call into the waiting room.

"Hey, baby, I got to go. I will be home soon. I love you," I said.

"I love you too. Bye, baby," Luke said quietly.

"Bye," I said, and I hung up the phone.

"Right this way," the nurse said with a cheesy smile as she led me toward my enemy, the scale.

I took off my shoes and tried to make myself as light as possible. I looked away as the nurse was balancing my weight.

"Could you please not tell me how much I weigh now?" I said. "I don't want to know until it had gone down instead of up."

The nurse looked at me and said, "One hundred and five pounds."

"Wow, that's amazing. I have lost weight since becoming pregnant!" I let out a sigh of relief as I realized the hardest part of my appointment was over.

I went into a small room and waited for the doctor. This was another doctor whom I didn't know. He came in and gave me a lecture about weight gain and the risk of diabetes. It took everything I had to hold back my tears that were always close to the surface.

We listened to Hayden's steady heartbeat, and once again I felt peace. With each *bump-bump* of his heartbeat, it was a reminder that God was giving us a miracle and he was the God of everything, including the decision Luke and I were facing.

Within ten minutes, my appointment was over, and I was happy to leave the doctor's office. I was sick of going to see a doctor. It seemed that about once a week there was an appointment for something. Most of the appointments were for Luke, and I really dreaded those.

I got into my car and let the tears flow. I could no longer contain my emotions. I looked down at my large stomach and thought about how I was six months along and had already exceeded my thirty-five-pound weight gain limit. I decided right then and there that I was not setting foot in another medical office again. I was so sick of how insensitive doctors could seem and how unimportant they made me feel.

I drove the short two miles home. I was unsure of how Luke would be acting, as he sounded upset on the phone. And who could blame him? He had been so positive throughout everything, he deserved to be upset now and then. I arrived and found Luke sitting in his green recliner chair watching TV.

"Hey, baby," I said as I entered the room.

"Hi, sweetie. How was your appointment?" Luke said.

"Terrible!" I replied quickly. "I don't know how much weight I have gained for sure, but it must be a lot because the doctor gave me a lecture about weight gain and everything. I don't know why I am gaining so much; I have been exercising a lot!" I said with tears forming in my eyes.

"Baby, don't worry about the weight gain. The important thing is that Hayden is healthy," Luke said as he reached for my hand. "And you still look beautiful!" Luke added.

Luke's tenderness touched me once again and made me smile. He was always thinking of me and was sensitive of my needs despite everything happening to him. Luke was right—the important thing was that Hayden was doing well. I decided to try not to compare myself with other women and ask people how much they gained during their pregnancy but be content with my ever-growing body.

Suddenly, I realized how selfish I was by focusing on my small problem of weight gain when Luke had an appointment as well, and we needed to talk about it.

"So, what did they tell you at your appointment?" I asked. Luke inhaled deeply and slowly let the air out. That was something he did whenever he was about to talk about something serious.

"Well, the doctor whom I went to see today was for a second opinion on whether I should do the amputation or keep my leg. He was a real jerk. It just seemed like he was trying to impress this intern girl who was there. He kept putting my x-rays up and discussing them with her. I didn't really learn anything from him today, except that I don't want to see him again!" Luke said.

"I'm sorry, baby," I said.

"How are you feeling about everything today?" I asked.

"I don't know. I have been praying about it and it is just such a difficult decision. I think I am kind of leaning toward saving my leg and removing the tumor from it. I just can't imagine my leg gone, ya know?"

"I know, baby. I think that is a good decision," I said and thought about how the tumor-removing surgery seemed to be a logical choice over the amputation. Just the word *amputation* made me uncomfortable. The thought of Luke having his leg cut off scared me. I was glad about the decision he was considering to make.

Later that night, while Luke and I were lying in bed, Luke's body began to tremble as he fought with all his might to keep back tears.

"Why, God?!" Luke yelled so intensely that it frightened me.

I stroked his face and found that he had been crying. Soon I was crying too.

"Why, God? Why do I have to make this decision?" Luke yelled as he finally voiced his pent-up emotions.

I continued stroking his face and wiping away his warm tears as my own tears fell on him.

"God, can't you see how much this is affecting everyone I love? Why God? Why? Can't you see I have a wife and a baby? I'm going to have a *baby*!" Luke said, his body fully heaving. He was gasping for air.

My mind was spinning. I felt as though I was in a nightmare—a nightmare in which you try and try to wake up but you never can. I didn't know what to do; I didn't know what to say. I continued to hold on tightly to Luke, and I echoed his prayer.

"Why, God?" I said in a near whisper.

Luke continued to let out his emotions. "God, I can handle this happening to me, but not how much it is hurting the ones I love. Why does everyone have to love me so much? Why does it have to hurt them so much?" Luke said.

I watched as every muscle in Luke's body tensed and stretched from head to toe, as if he was trying to break out of his body. I trembled in fear, as I had never seen these emotions from my husband and did not know what to do to calm him down.

"It's okay, baby," I said in between sobs. "It's okay, it's okay," I repeated over and over.

God? Are you there? I prayed silently. *Please God, give me the words to say, show me how to help Luke. I can't do this on my own, I really need you right now.* Please*!* I cried out silently.

Luke's body continued to heave in and out. I was overwhelmed by Luke's sudden flood of emotions. Before this time, I was not aware of what was going on inside of him. Minutes passed and Luke continued to cry. As I laid my head on his chest and continued to pray to God for wisdom and strength, Luke's sobs became softer and less frequent.

With my head on Luke's chest, I listened to the sound of his heartbeat. My head rose and fell with every breath that he took, and I sensed that he was beginning to calm down.

"I love you, baby," Luke said in a near whisper.

"I love you too," I replied.

"Can I pray for you?" I asked.

"Yes."

I closed my eyes and talked to the one and only peace giver. "Dear Jesus, we need you so very much right now." My tears were now heavily flowing onto Luke's chest. "We thank you for giving us each other, God. I thank you so much for Luke. I love him so much. We have a big decision to make. I pray that you will give us peace about the decision and help us to know for sure what you want us to do. We can't do this without you, we are lost without you. God, we don't understand why this is happening, but we trust you. You have the greater plan. Help us to know what to do. Please God, give Luke peace. Help him to rest tonight and know that you will take care of us. We love you, Jesus. Amen."

Luke continued to hold me and cry with me. I felt an indescribable peace come over me. It was a peace that could not be put into words because there was not a word that would do justice to what it was like. I felt that God had scooped me up in his arms and was holding me close to his heart.

I made a decision that night that I was no longer going to let anger be a part of my reaction to what was happening to Luke. Anger was not something that was going to make anything better. It would do the opposite. It would sit inside of me like rotten milk, making everything it came into contact with smell sour. I did not want to be angry anymore. Satan wanted me to be angry. God wanted to give me his indescribable peace and take away my rotting milk, my anger. As the peace continued to cover me, I fell asleep in Luke's arms.

The next day, I kissed Luke good-bye as I left for work. As I drove, I thought about the emotions I had seen from Luke. I was glad that he had finally let his emotions out rather than keep them inside. I knew that Luke was trying to be strong for me, but it was good for me to see his real emotions and his honesty before God and myself. I realized that we were still facing an incredibly hard decision, but I felt God's peace covering me, and I had the strength to make it through another day.

I considered the options before us again. Neither one sounded very good to me. I couldn't imagine Luke on crutches for a whole year and then wearing a special boot for the rest of his life. On the other hand, I couldn't imagine Luke having his leg amputated. Luke had always been so active and into sports. I thought back to a spring day in 1996…

"Hey, Rommel, are you coming to the game today?" Luke playfully asked me, calling me by my last name at that time.

"As long as you wear those cute baseball pants!" I replied in a flirting tone.

"Okay," Luke replied as he walked out the door of our home ec class.

"See you later," I said with a smile. I was planning to watch our high school's baseball team play after school.

Luke and I had gotten to know each other in our home economics class. I wasn't that into baseball, but I enjoyed sitting in the sun, talking with friends, and looking at cute boys, so baseball had all the elements I needed.

"Hey, Shelly, are you coming?" One of my best friends Lana said to me. Lana was my only friend who went to sports games to actually pay attention to the game and not the boys.

"Ya, just a second," I said as I closed my locker.

We walked across the field to where the baseball game was being played. It was a warm sunny day and I was excited to be outside. We sat down on the bleachers and watched the game. I looked through the metal fence and saw that Luke was up to bat.

"He sure is cute," I said to Lana.

"Who?" Lana replied, totally involved in the game.

"Luke Bader," I said with a smile. I thought he was cute but wasn't interested in dating him, as one of my friends had already dated him. I would never want to break the "code." There was an unwritten rule between us girls, that you never dated anyone's ex-boyfriend or someone whom they were interested in. That made things a little difficult sometimes since we went to a small private school.

I watched in amazement as Luke was able to hit the first ball that was pitched him. *Crack!* went the bat. The ball flew through the air and continued to fly farther and farther away.

"Home run!" I heard several people yell.

"Way to go, Bader!" I yelled and joined in the crowd's cheering. Luke ran quickly around the bases and back to home plate.

Soon it was our turn to be in the field, and I watched as Luke took his place on the pitching mound. I could see that he was secretly communicating with the pitcher. He threw the first pitch.

"Strike," the umpire called out.

Luke took the ball in his left hand and prepared to pitch it again. The ball flew out of his hand.

"Strike," the umpire called again.

Once more, Luke took the ball in his hand and threw it with amazing force and speed.

"Strike three," the umpire called out.

The crowd once again cheered, and it was evident to all that Luke was truly the star of the team.

As I pulled into the parking lot at work, I was saddened to think of the choice that was now before the star player. Once again, I asked the LORD to give us peace.

"God, show us what to do." I pleaded and waited for an answer.

Back to Hotel Sunnyside

❧❧❧

The days continued to pass, and we still had not made a decision about Luke's leg. We had to continue on with Luke's chemo treatment. I was not looking forward to going back to "Hotel Sunnyside." It hadn't been that bad the last time, but it had a very distinct smell that always made me feel nauseous.

I had already made plans for my substitute and was off work in order to stay with Luke in the hospital. The day of the treatment arrived, and we headed to see Luke's oncologist. This time, Luke had to see the oncologist first, and then the oncologist would put in the order for his chemo in the hospital.

As we entered the sterile medical office, I felt sick to my stomach. I never looked forward to seeing other cancer patients in the waiting room. All the bare heads were a reminder of the sickness overtaking so many people's bodies. We were called back to the oncology room and waited for Luke's oncologist.

I looked around the small room and felt like I was suffocating. With every crinkle of the paper where Luke was sitting, I felt as though I would faint. The door slowly creaked open. A tall, lanky doctor with thick glassed walked into the room.

"Hi, Luke," the doctor said with no emotion visible on his face.

"Hi," Luke replied with an equal lack of emotion in his voice.

"Well, how are you feeling today?" the doctor asked.

"Okay," Luke replied.

As they were talking, I wondered how many people this doctor had seen die. I thought he had a depressing job, one that I could never do. He seemed so insensitive to Luke and made me feel as though I was invisible. I was just another crying wife, which he had seen hundreds of time. He seemed to be so desensitized to the person whom cancer was affecting. I wondered if anyone he loved had ever had cancer. I listened once again to their conversation.

"Well, Luke, you can go to Sunnyside tomorrow morning, but there is no guarantee you will get a bed. Or you can go and try to get one tonight and go ahead and get the chemo started," the doctor said.

Luke looked at me. "Let's get it over with and start tonight."

"That's a good idea," I said.

I was glad that we had already packed and had everything we needed in the car. We left the medical office and proceeded to drive to the hospital. We were soon parked and entering "Hotel Sunnyside." I found it more difficult to carry all of my things into the hospital as compared to the last time.

Automatic doors greeted us in the entrance of the hospital where we would be staying for the next five days. I crossed the threshold from my world into the hospital and felt instantly nauseous. Our feet made a loud *clomp* with every step we took and echoed throughout the halls. We made our way to the admittance room. There was a woman busily looking over papers at a small desk covered with books and pencils. She looked up from what she was doing.

"May I help you?" she said while setting down her pen.

"Yes, I am here for my chemo treatment," Luke said.

"Okay, what is your name?"

"Luke Bader."

The woman quickly began typing on her computer. "You are in room 103," she said. "Here is the phone number." She handed it to me. She didn't realize I was staying with him. I guess it was kind of rare for a wife to stay with her husband for five days in the hospital, especially a pregnant wife!

We left the office with all of our bags and headed down the long hallway to the oncology wing of the hospital. As we came closer to room 103, we were greeted by several nurses who remembered Luke. As we passed the private room we had stayed in the first time, I wondered what kind of room we would be living in this time. We walked almost completely to the end of the hall and found a door with the numbers 103 next to it. There was an elderly couple in the room. A thin, frail woman was lying on the bed with an older man beside her. I thought there was a mistake in the room we were given, but I looked farther and saw that past a dividing curtain, by the window, was a small bed. We entered the room.

"Hi," I said quietly as we passed the elderly couple.

I heard a faint hi in reply.

We made our way over to the bed. The room felt very hot and stuffy. I looked around and realized that there was not even a bed or any possible space for me to stay. I felt very disappointed and tried to hold back my tears. Luke sat down on the bed, and I began to put away our things in the small closet that was provided. I looked at Luke's face and knew that he, too, was disappointed about the room that had been given to us. I knew he was hoping for a private room again.

"Do you think there are any other rooms available?" I said in a whisper, as not to disturb our roommates on the other side of the thin curtain barrier.

"I don't know, but I hope so. This is too small, and there is no room for you to sleep." Luke said.

"I know. When the nurse comes in, lets ask." I said, as I found a small chair to sit down in. A few minutes passed and a nurse walked in.

"Hi, I am here to get your IV going," she said matter of factly. I was unfamiliar with the nurse. She did not seem very friendly.

"We were wondering if there are any other rooms available. I am planning on staying all four nights with him, and it doesn't look like there is room for me to stay here," I said.

The nurse looked at me kind of funny, as if I was crazy for wanting to stay with my husband in the hospital. "We are really busy right now, but I can check if there is anything available. I will be back in just a minute," She quickly walked out of the room.

I could hear muffled voices coming from the other side of the room, and I wondered what they were talking about. I wondered what kind of cancer the woman next to Luke had. Was it terminal? Did the chemo help her? Did her husband stay with her? I often wondered what other people's cancer stories were.

I heard footsteps entering the room. I looked up and saw my parents walking in.

"Hi," my mom said.

"Hi," I replied. "Can you believe how tiny this room is? We just asked if we could get a different one, and a nurse is going to come back and tell us if we can in a few minutes," I said.

My parents looked around our half of the tiny room.

"Yeah, it's pretty tight in here," my dad said.

"Here, you can have this chair," I told my mom as I got up and sat down on the bed with Luke. Even with my dad standing, the four of us barely fit in the room. I noticed that Luke was dripping sweat from his face. Luke was easily hot and sweaty. The stuffy room was making "Hotel Sunnyside" almost unbearable for him.

I said a silent prayer for Luke:

Dear God, please help us to get in another room. It would be so much easier for Luke if we had more space and a cooler room. I pray that by some miracle there will be an open bed somewhere. Thanks. Amen.

The nurse entered the room. "I found a bed for you. It isn't a private room, but it is bigger and will have room for your wife to sleep," the nurse said. I whispered a prayer of thanks.

I began gathering up our items out of the closet. I put as many bags as I could hold on my shoulders and tried to balance them. My protruding stomach made it difficult to balance, but I did the best that I could. I was happy that my parents were there to help us move our things. After all of our things were gathered, we followed the nurse back down to the other end of the hall. She showed us the room we would now be staying in. Seeing our new room, I could tell that it was about three times larger than the previous one.

We were going to be staying on the right side of the room. I looked to the left side and was saddened by what I saw. Lying on the small hospital bed was a man who appeared to be sleeping. I looked closer and saw that he was very thin. I could tell that in his precancer days, he was a man of average build and size. His brown skin now looked as though it was barely hanging onto his bones. His side of the room was decorated with flowers, cards, and balloons. There was a large card that I could tell was made by children. It said "We miss you" and was signed by many kids. I wondered what kind of work he did with kids.

My heart fell into a deeper sadness as I saw that he did not have anyone sitting by his side. I wondered where his family was. Did he have a wife? Kids? Where were they? I could not imagine not being by my husband's side through every day of treatment that he had to endure.

Luke went to his new bed, and I knew he was anxious to get his treatment started so that he could get it over with. I once again began unpacking our things. I found that there was a chair which turned into a bed for me. I was pleased to see that it was a larger bed than the last time we stayed in the hospital.

"Okay Luke, let's get your IV started," the nurse said as soon as Luke was in his new bed.

Throughout the evening, Luke's visitors continued to come in. Every once in a while, we would hear a moan from the other side of the room, and I couldn't help wondering what was happening to the man we were sharing a room with.

When it was time for bed, I began my pre-bed routines. I folded out the little bed I would be sleeping on. I put down a foam pad as well as a body pillow. I kissed Luke goodnight and tried to make myself comfortable. The *swish*, *pump*, *swish*, *pump* sounds of Luke's IV continued to go. As I lay down, I found it hard to sleep as there was light peeking its way through the blinds. I got up and readjusted them. They still didn't keep the light out, but I knew there was nothing I could do about it.

I finally relaxed and tried to forget where I was. I closed my eyes and began to drift off to sleep.

"*Ah!*" a loud voice yelled.

I was quickly awakened and reminded of where I was. The lights were instantly turned on, and I could hear the voices of the nurses. I realized that something was very wrong with the man behind the curtain.

Luke and I looked at each other. I said a silent prayer for the man. A few minutes later, the lights were turned off and I tried to sleep again. The moaning came again, and it grew louder. Again, the lights were turned on and there were more words from the nurses that I couldn't make out. This continued throughout the whole night. Luke and I didn't get very much sleep that night. It was very disturbing physically and emotionally. Hearing this man's cries made cancer even more of a reality to me. He was in so much pain, and there was nothing that anyone could do about it. My hate for cancer grew that night. I began to visualize that cancer was an evil beast, and I wanted to strangle it to death and then it could never come back to destroy anyone's life again. I felt tired, I felt angry and most of all, I felt scared— scared for the future of my husband's life. I prayed and prayed that the evil cancer beast would never destroy the body of my one true love, my sweet husband.

I drifted in and out of sleep and tried to take my mind to another place. I needed a memory of a happier time to help me escape the reality of my present situation. As I closed my eyes, fuzzy images began to come into focus, and I could hear the sound of laughter.

"Look, he's going to do it!" I yelled enthusiastically as I peered out the window of my parents' house.

I was instantly joined by my mom and my two sisters-in-law, Jessica and Amy. The four of us peeked through the window and watched as my dad and Luke walked outside to where my dad was going to feed the cows. The beautiful landscape of the countryside was a perfect place for Luke to ask my dad for my hand in marriage.

I quickly grabbed my video camera in an effort to preserve the moment that I wanted to one day show my children.

"Oh, that is so cute," Jessica said.

"How do you know he is asking him right now?" Amy asked.

"Well, I know he is going to ask me soon, and why else would he ask to go take a walk with dad? You know he isn't much of a talker!" I replied.

"Neither is your dad," my mom said as she smiled brightly with a hint of tears brimming in her eyes.

I continued looking outside and saw the two most important men in the world to me. That moment was the first time I realized how alike they were. My dad had always been the strong, silent type who didn't always let me know what he was thinking. He was always a very good provider and made sure we knew that we were loved. He reminded me of a rock. When he talked, we listened and obeyed. Dad's word was final. There was nothing in the world that could make him falter from his convictions and faith in God. Inside that rock, there was also a soft layer of emotions that could be seen from time to time. I have always enjoyed those occasional glimpses into the softer layer.

Luke also possessed the characteristics that my dad did. He was strong like a rock. His soft layer was a mystery to everyone else, but not to me. As I looked at him, I realized that he would probably keep his soft layer hidden from our children. I thought about what Luke had told me one time. He had said that while he was like a rock, I was like a stock market, you never knew if I was going to be up or down!

I put down the video camera and continued with the Thanksgiving preparations. I was trying to become "wifely" since I knew marriage was in the near future, so I had baked several apple pies. Luke was so proud of me but complained that I made a mess.

I watched the rock of my past and the rock of my future walk toward the house, and I thanked God that I was so extremely blessed.

The bright lights jolted me from my memories and brought me back to the pain of the present. I felt hot tears beginning to moisten my eyes as I fought with all my strength to hold them back. It was my turn to be the rock, my turn to be strong.

Suddenly, I felt as though God was whispering in my ear, whispering words that I had not thought of in a long time. I heard them and knew they were a special gift for me.

"Michelle, I am the rock, your fortress, and your deliverer; I am your rock in whom you take refuge. I am your shield and the horn of your salvation, your stronghold" (Psalm 18:2).

"Oh, God." I prayed silently. "Thank you for being the rock; I cannot do it alone! I am scared."

I paused to look at my husband who was resting his eyes and probably doing the same thing as me. I could now taste salt from my tears as I struggled to keep my crying muffles. I did not want to bother Luke.

"Jesus," I continued, "This is bigger than anything I have ever been through. Please show me what to do to be an encouragement and help to my husband. Help me to continue to let go of the anger. I can feel it trying to take its place in my life, and I don't want it! God, please once again give me your indescribable peace and also give it to Luke. I thank you for him. I thank you for his positive attitude. Thank you that through him, others can see you. Oh, LORD, we are still facing such a big decision with Luke's leg. Please give us direction about whether to do the amputation or not. Thank you for promising that you will not give us more than we can handle. Thank you for being my peace and my rock."

I kept my eyes closed, and the lights soon turned off. A peace soon fell over me and I fell fast asleep.

When I woke up in the morning, I felt peace but I still felt torn about the decision that continued to linger over us every day. It was not an easy choice and I didn't know how we were ever going to decide.

One day at a time, I said to myself as I prepared to speak to Luke about the decision.

Sleepless Nights

❧❀❧

I knew it was time for Luke and I to make a final decision about his leg, but I truly had no idea what we were going to do. How do you make that kind of decision? I stared at Luke's swollen ankle through sleep-filled eyes. I could see that Luke's tumor was now protruding from his bone and had the appearance of a swollen ankle. I thought back to the time he told me it was bothering him.

❧❀❧

"We're almost there," I said, starting to lose my breath.

I looked down and saw how far up we now were. We had been hiking for quite some time now on a narrow winding path.

"Hey Luke, this looks like a great place for a picture," I said as I excitedly ran to look closer. I looked in awe at the cascading waterfall behind me. It gave off a soft mist that felt refreshing on my face.

"Another picture?" Luke replied. "Don't we have enough?"

"I just want to remember every moment I am with you," I said excitedly. I looked at Luke and couldn't wait to be his wife. Only eighty-two more days to go! From the day we got engaged, I kept track of how many more days it would be until I would be Luke's wife.

"Excuse me, would you mind taking a picture for us?" I requested to an older gentleman coming on the path toward us.

"Sure. Do I just push this button?" he asked.

"Yes," I said as I walked toward Luke and wrapped my arms around him as he did the same to me. We smiled our best posed smiles.

Luke and I, hand in hand, continued up the trail. When the trail became very narrow, we had to let go of each others hands. I felt safe with Luke next to me. I knew that he would do everything in his power to keep me from harm. The trail continued to get steeper. Luke stopped walking and looked down.

"What's wrong?" I asked.

"It's my ankle again, it is really hurting."

"You really should go to a doctor to get that checked out," I said. I wondered what it could be. It seemed to me that it was a sprained ankle or something of the sort.

"I think I will soon," Luke said as he bent down to take a closer look. With sweat dripping down his face, he stood up and looked at me. I couldn't help thinking once again how handsome he was. His deep-brown eyes were complemented by his tanned skin and dark-brown hair. He had such an amazing strong presence about him. He was strong mentally and physically.

Luke and I joined hands and completed our hike to the top of the picturesque Multnomah Falls.

"Oh, it is so beautiful!" I cried excitedly. I stood as close to the edge of the rail as possible and watched the water fall to the ground. It fell forcefully yet gracefully.

The mist once again felt refreshing on my face. Waterfalls had always been one of my favorite natural wonders. I breathed in slowly and gazed at the beauty before me.

Luke walked up behind me and put his arms around my waist. I could feel his breath on my neck and the rhythm of his heart on my back. We stood in silence and enjoyed the moment.

I, of course, had to take the camera back out. I snapped some pictures of Luke and then we posed together as I stretched my arm out as far as it could go in order to try to get a picture of us together. I also held out my hand with my beautiful engagement ring and took a picture with the water as a cascading background.

"What are you doing?" Luke said with a curious look on his face.

"Just admiring my ring and taking a picture of it with the waterfall," I said.

I was always taking pictures of everything important to me. The ring was an important symbol of the vow I would soon make. The waterfall was something I also wanted to capture and keep in my memory. I had been to that waterfall several times before, but it never seemed so beautiful as the day I went there with Luke. It was the kind of romantic setting that I had always seen myself and my "dream man" in. It was nice to be sharing that dream with my real-life man.

We hiked back down the trail, and I could tell by the look on Luke's face that he was in pain. Luke was never one to tell me that he was in pain. I, on the other hand, would tell him of every little headache or sickness I was feeling.

"Is your ankle still bothering you?" I asked as we made our way to the car.

"Yes," Luke said. "Tomorrow I will make an appointment."

"Good," I replied.

Soon after that day, Luke went to see a doctor. He was told that it was tendonitis, and he was given medication. At the time, I was relieved to hear that it was nothing serious. Looking back now, it is hard not to be angry.

My eyes filled with tears as I looked again at Luke's swollen ankle. *Swish, pump, swish, pump,* the chemo continued. I wondered if the first doctor who had seen Luke would have diagnosed him correctly, would we still have to make an amputation decision? Would finding the cancer earlier have made any difference? As I thought about these things, I could feel my enemy—my anger—trying to take control of me again. My enemy wanted me to hate the doctor, to be bitter about cancer, to be jealous of others, to not be at peace, and to destroy myself with the constant what ifs and whys.

I pondered the timing of everything. If Luke had been diagnosed with cancer in June, would the wedding have gone on as planned? With all my heart I still would have wanted to marry him, but would he marry me? He had once told me that he wished I had never married him so he could have saved me so much pain and heartache. I told him that I would rather have pain and heartache with him then be anywhere without him.

It was not until six months later that he was diagnosed. I looked down at my barely recognizable stomach, and I continued thinking about God's amazing timing.

"Hayden," I whispered softly.

What an amazing gift God had given us. In the midst of all the challenges facing us, he had given us the gift of life. Luke had always said we were going to wait three to five years before having a baby. I, on the other hand, wanted one as soon as possible. We had compromised by saying we could wait two years. Unlike our plan, two months into our marriage we had our lovely surprise pregnancy!

As I continued looking at Luke, I wondered how many more things in my life God would have the perfect timing. I always thought I knew the best timing for everything, but God knew better.

Luke looked up from the paper he was reading. "How are your emotions today?" Luke said. He was always so sensitive to how I was feeling both physically and emotionally. He could easily read how I was doing by a simple glance at my face. I wasn't good at hiding my emotions, especially from him.

"Okay," I replied as my eyes fell to the floor. "I have been praying, and I still don't know what we should do! Are you thinking of the amputation or cutting the tumor out?"

"I don't know, baby, and honestly, I don't want to think about it right now," Luke said. I could tell by the tone of his voice that the chemo was beginning to wear on him. He looked tired. I decided to drop the subject for the time being. I hated not knowing the future. I didn't know which decision we were going to make, or how we would ever decide.

As the day wore on, I could see how tired Luke was becoming. I felt exhausted as well. I didn't think that I could physically or emotionally handle another night in that hospital room. I thought back to the moaning from the other side of the room from the night before. I did not want to leave Luke by himself, but I really, truly didn't think I could go another night in the same circumstance as the night before.

"Luke," I said as I turned to face my husband in the small hospital room.

"Yes," Luke said, stretching his hand out to reach mine. I took his hand in my own.

"I don't know if I can stay here another night" Tears formed in my eyes. "I want to be with you, but I need rest." I rubbed my stomach.

"I know, sweetie. I want you to stay at home tonight. I will be okay," Luke said softly.

"Are you sure?" I asked.

"Yes, it is what is best for you and Hayden," Luke replied as a smile came across his face at the mention of Hayden.

"Okay," I said as I got up to start packing some of my things.

It was such a difficult decision to leave my husband's side, but I knew I needed to give my body and my baby rest that would not come from another sleepless night in the hospital.

"Well, I guess I will go. I hope you sleep better tonight. I love you so very much," I said as I kissed Luke good-bye.

"I love you too," Luke said as I turned to leave.

As I began the walk to the car, my heart sank. Was I making the right decision? Guilt took over my entire body as I passed room after room of cancer patients. Why can I get to go home and sleep in my warm cozy bed (or my marshmallow, as Luke and I call it) while these people had to stay in their sterile rooms getting pumped full of poison?

God, I don't understand you, but I trust you, I said silently as I got into my car.

As I started the engine, my tears could no longer be suppressed. All the emotions that I had tried to keep inside in order to be strong for Luke made their way out in the form of warm, salty tears.

I wiped my eyes and began to drive home. The cold air was making me shiver, so I reached to turn on the heater. I tuned in the radio to the Christian station. I needed comfort, and I knew God was the one to give it to me. My tears turned into sobs as I heard the sounds of the song "It Is Well with My Soul." The words spoke to me so directly that I knew they were a message from my Savior to me.

When peace, like a river, attendeth my way,
When sorrows like sea billows roll;
Whatever my lot, thou hast taught me to say,
It is well, it is well with my soul.

"LORD, help me to realize that this is the plan you have for us," I prayed through tears.

It is well with my soul;
It is well, it is well with my soul.

I sang the words through the sobs.

Though Satan should buffet, though trials should come,
Let this blest assurance control,
That Christ has regarded my helpless estate,
And has shed his own blood for my soul.

"Jesus," I prayed fervently. "Thank you for shedding your blood, thank you for the cross, thank you for your plan, and thank you, most of all, that I can rest assure that you have the best plans in store for Luke and I."

My sin—O the bliss of this glorious thought!—
My sin, not in part, but the whole,
Is nailed to the cross and I bear it no more;
Praise the LORD, praise the LORD, O my soul!

"Thank you, Jesus, for taking away my sins and making me into the person you created me to be. You created me to be Luke's wife, and you know this time

in our life would come, and you have not left us alone.
Thank you that even in the midst of all of this, I can
still feel your presence," I prayed.

> O LORD, haste the day when the faith shall be
> sight,
> The clouds be rolled back as a scroll,
> The trump shall resound and the LORD shall
> descend;
> "Even so"—it is well with my soul.
>
> —Horatio Gates Spafford

"Oh, Jesus, one day you will come back for us, and
none of this will matter anymore. We will be with you,
and Luke will be healthy, and the trials of the world
will be so far away. Thank you for putting things into
perspective for me. You are so awesome, and I truly
love you and thank you for all the wonderful things you
have given me," I prayed as the song ended.

After crying and praying, I felt better. I felt as
though a weight had been lifted from me. I thought of
the story of Horatio Gates Spafford, the man who had
written the song. He wrote the song while on a ship
over the place where his four daughters had died. If he
could write the words "It is well with my soul" while
looking over the place where his daughters had passed
away, then I could say that it was well with my soul in
my present circumstance.

I parked the car in the garage and walked into my
house. It was strange knowing that it would be empty. I
entered the dark living room and quickly turned on the
lights. Somehow I felt less alone if the lights were on.

I got ready for bed and shut and locked our bedroom door, which was something I never did when Luke was there. In the seven months that we were married, I had never spent a night at our house without Luke.

I turned out the lights and quickly climbed into our "marshmallow." The coolness of the sheets made me shiver, and the usual body heat of Luke was not there to warm me up. I thought of Luke and wondered how he was doing. There was an empty feeling in the house, and I didn't like it. It was strange to be sleeping on our bed without him. And it was even stranger for me to think of Luke lying on a small bed with uncomfortable blankets and pillows and a needle in his arm.

"God, please be with Luke right now," I whispered as I closed my eyes and let my overwhelming tiredness take over. I quickly drifted off to sleep.

My eyes fluttered open, and I instinctively reached for Luke. The empty space reminded me that Luke was still in the hospital, and I was alone. I quickly got out of bed so that I could shower and return to Luke as fast as possible.

Within an hour, I was back in the hospital and walking into Luke's room where he was eating breakfast—eggs covered in ketchup.

"Hi, baby," I said as I walked into the room.

"Hey," Luke replied.

"How was your night?"

"Depressing, very depressing. I don't ever want to spend another night here without you. I didn't get much sleep, and I missed you," Luke said.

"I missed you too. I am sorry I was gone, but I feel more refreshed and I won't leave you again," I said as I kissed him softly.

"It was so depressing just lying here with no one beside me. I can't imagine it being like that all the time. I just wanted you to be next to me," Luke said.

"I am really sorry. I promise, I will not leave you again," I said, feeling more guilty than ever for leaving him alone.

This is what it is all about, I thought. *Marriage. For better or for worse, in sickness and in health.* We were living it. We were living our vows. I decided right then and there that no matter what, I would rather have a million sleepless nights next to Luke than one restful night all alone.

Crushed in Spirit

I endured two more pretty much sleepless nights with Luke in the hospital. Both nights were as eventful as the first two. On the third day, we moved to a private room which we enjoyed for about an hour, and then we were told we had to move back to the room we had come for. I was very tired and my body ached from the trips up and down the hall with all of our things. I looked down at my swollen feet, and for a second I felt sorry for myself.

What do other pregnant women have to complain about? I thought bitterly. *This isn't fair!* I quickly reminded myself that this was God's plan for my life, and he would never put me through more than I could handle.

After we were settled back in our room, a nurse entered.

"I know you guys just moved, but we have a room that is private for now and you can move into it if you want," she said.

I looked at Luke and I already knew his answer.

"Yes, we will do it," I said as I picked up our bags for what seemed like the hundredth time. We walked down the hall once again and entered the last room in the hall on the left hand side. It was larger than the last room and had two beds, which were both empty. Luke walked to the one closest to the window. His IV post squeaked as the wheels rolled on the smooth surface of the floor. Luke proceeded to sit down on the bed while I began putting our things away for what I hoped would be the last time.

My attention was suddenly drawn to the room across ours. I heard the all-too-familiar sound of crying. I saw a girl who looked like she was about sixteen, She had a blue scarf on her head, and I knew she had been undergoing chemotherapy. I didn't like seeing a teenager like that. I thought back to my own carefree teenage years and was thankful that I had been healthy and full of life. I don't know how I would have handled cancer at such a young age. Her cries tore at my already sensitive heart. I said a quick prayer for her.

Luke finished the rest of his chemo, and we were ready to go home. It was nice to be home and away from everything in the hospital. The decision we had to make still loomed over our heads. Luke and I had been praying about it everyday, and we finally felt that we had come to a decision.

Luke called the surgeon the next day to tell her about our choice. I listened as Luke talked.

"We have decided that we would like to do the bone-saving operation," Luke said as I thought about how it made more sense to save his leg than amputate.

"Uh-huh," Luke said while the surgeon spoke on the other end. I strained to hear what was being said, but the voice of the surgeon was too quiet.

"I understand," Luke said with a somber look on his face.

"Ya, she is right here," Luke said as he muffled the phone.

"She wants to talk to you." Luke handed the phone over to me. It took me by surprise that she wanted to speak to me.

"Hello," I said.

"Hi, I just want to talk to you about a couple of things."

"Okay," I replied, having no idea what to expect.

"I just want you guys to think about the decision some more. I really recommend doing the amputation. I know it sounds extreme, but I really think that it would be the way for Luke to maintain an active lifestyle. There is also less of a chance of the tumor reoccurring because we would cut it all out and leave a very big margin. I know it is a hard choice, but I think Luke would have a hard time with the other surgery. He would have to wear a boot the rest of his life. With the amputation, he would be able to walk a few months after surgery and would one day be able to run and play sports again. Without amputation, Luke will never be able to do those things again. And his health is really the most important thing. If we did the bone-saving surgery and the tumor was to ever come back, we would have to do an above-the-knee amputation. Above-the-knee is much harder to adjust to."

I listened intently trying to take in all of this information. Her words made sense. *Amputation* was just such a big, scary word. I never thought we would ever have to make a decision like this.

My hand was shaking as I tried to steady the phone to my ear. My eyes began to blur as warm tears overflowed onto my cheeks. My mind was spinning at the new information I had just been given. Before talking to the surgeon, I was mentally preparing myself for the bone-saving surgery. I did not want to have to prepare myself to the even more extreme alternative—amputation.

I realized that I had been silent for a while and I needed to resume my conversation. "I understand what you are saying," I said quietly. "We will think about it and get back to you."

"All right. The sooner you make the decision, the better. We will talk soon," said the surgeon.

"Okay, bye," I said as I hung up the phone. I looked at Luke. He had his index finger pressed against his lip, and his eyebrows were tight and close together. I knew instantly that he was deep in thought. I walked up to him and wrapped my arms around his strong body. Having him near me made me feel a little better. We stood in silence for a few minutes, both of us deep in our own thoughts.

"So, what do you think now?" I said as I broke the silence.

Luke inhaled deeply and slowly exhaled. "I think we should keep praying about it." His answer was short and simple, and I knew he needed time to think about it. Luke was never one to make quick decisions. He always researched things thoroughly before making a decision, and I knew this time would not be different.

Though Luke and I had only been married eight months, I had learned many things about my husband. I knew that he needed time to be alone and pray and process things on his own. He would talk to me when he was ready, and I would not push the issue until he brought it up.

I left my husband alone and dealt with this the way that was best for me. I immediately called my mom. As I dialed her number, I thought back to the many conversations I had with her regarding who would one day be my husband. I reflected on her wisdom and prayed that one day I could even be half the woman she was. I let my mind continue to wander into the far past of my teenage years...

"It's not okay, Mom. I will never let myself care for someone again!" I said as I gasped for air in between my heaving sobs. My young sixteen-year-old heart had never known such pain.

My mom held me in her lap as I cried the tears that could only come from a broken heart. She continued to stroke my hair gently and reminded me what she had told me so many times before.

"God is just protecting you from the wrong ones. I have been praying for your future husband since you were in my womb. I know it hurts, but God does have a plan for your life."

I heard her words, but it did not stop the intense pain I was feeling. The feelings of rejection and abandonment overtook my mind. I never wanted to be hurt again. I wanted it to go away. It seemed there was nothing I could do to dull the pain in my young heart. My sobs continued as I reminded myself of my present situation and how my heart had been broken.

"Michelle, I know that it is difficult now, but someday you will look back on this and it will not hurt anymore. God and time are the best healers of a broken heart. In fact, there is a verse I want to share with you; it has meant a lot to me. When my mom—your grandmother—passed away, I found this verse to be of great comfort to me.

"The LORD is close to the brokenhearted and saves those who are crushed in spirit" (Psalm 34:18).

I let God's holy words find their way into my broken heart and begin to heal my heart. I never forgot those words. There were many times that I was brokenhearted and crushed in spirit, and God would speak those words to me in his way that is too personal and breathtaking to describe. *Brokenhearted, brokenhearted, brokenhearted*…I repeated those words over and over as I waited for my mom's voice at the other end of the phone.

"Hello," my mom said quietly.

"Hi, it's me," I said.

"What's wrong?" My mom knew in an instant that I was upset.

"I just don't know what we are going to do now," I said as I strained to hold back my tears. "The surgeon called, and she said she thinks that the amputation would be the best decision for Luke. I just can't imagine him without his leg, Mom! Why is this happening to him?" The tears were now freely flowing, and my body was now heaving from the strain of trying to hold back the tears. I gasped for air and tried to remind myself to breathe.

"Michelle, I am so sorry. I wish I could take away all the pain and make it better for you. Remember all the times we have talked about God having a plan for you? Well, this is it. This is God's plan. You were made to be Luke's wife. You were made to be with him at this very moment and support him in whatever decision he makes. God knew before you were born that you would be able to handle this. Remember, God will never give us more than we can handle. That means that God knows you can handle this."

I was comforted once again by the sound of my mom's voice and the wisdom she had once again imparted to me. We talked for a few more minutes, and she helped me feel better about things. After I hung up the phone, I walked into the living room and saw that Luke was sitting on the recliner appearing to read the newspaper, but I knew that his mind was not on current events. I walked into our bedroom. I closed the blinds and shut the curtains. I wanted to be alone. I wanted to shut out the light from the outside world—the world that did not have to deal with cancer or amputation. I threw myself on the bed and let all the emotion that I hid so many times from so many people cascade from my weak and tired body. I cried tears that were from a deeper broken heart than I had ever felt. I felt as though I could not breathe or speak or move. I felt crushed. My body, mind, and spirit were crushed. I closed my eyes and tried to pray, but there were no words. There were no words to express what I was feeling.

"Michelle, I am close to you." The words came softly like a smooth summer breeze. I realized that God was reminding me in his own way what he had told me before. He was with me and he was close to me—the me that was brokenhearted and crushed in spirit.

I continued to cry and release my emotions to God. I heard the door open, and I looked up to see Luke walking toward me.

"Baby," Luke said with deep concern in his voice.

He lay down next to me and held me close. My sobs grew louder. He said no words but let me continue crying until I calmed down. I listened once again to the calming beat of his heartbeat and felt safe once again. In his arms, I felt a comfort that could not be found from any other person. God gave him the special gift of being my flesh and blood comforter. God was my biggest comfort, but holding on to my husband was second best.

"I think we should do the amputation," Luke said suddenly.

"I know," I said with tears in my eyes.

Luke had been strong for me and now it was his turn to release his hidden inner emotions. His body began to tense, and I knew what was coming. I could see him straining with everything in me to hold back his pain-filled tears.

"It's okay," I said as I stroked his smooth face. Gone were the days of feeling scruff on his face, thanks to the chemo he had received. Then Luke began to cry a cry so filled with pain that it nearly took my breath away.

"Why, God? Why do I have to make this choice? I am only twenty-six! I don't want to lose my leg!" Luke cried out to God. The heaving continued. I had seen this emotion from my husband before and was more prepared for it this time.

"God," I prayed aloud. "Please comfort Luke. This is such a hard thing to have to do. We know you have a plan, but we do not see it at this moment. Give us peace and clarity." My head lay on Luke's chest and moved up and down with every anguish-filled breath Luke took. "Jesus," I continued, "Help us to feel a peace if we are supposed to do the amputation."

I continued to hold Luke and let him cry until there were no more tears left. I fell asleep in the peace and comfort of his arms and knew that somehow we could get through this.

A few days went by, and Luke and I continued to pray about what to do. I knew in my head what we should do, but my heart did not want it. I knew the best and smartest decision for Luke and our growing family was to do the amputation. I began to redirect my thinking and prepared myself for what lay ahead.

Together, Luke and I made our final decision: we would go ahead with the amputation. We began telling friends and family. The surgeon wanted to do it as soon as possible to get the cancer out, so the amputation was scheduled three weeks from the time we made the decision.

There are a lot of thoughts that go through your head when you know in a few weeks the one that you love will be losing a limb. What would Luke's emotions be like after the surgery? How would he adapt physically and mentally? Would he be angry? These were all unanswered questions that I would have to wait to find out.

We were supported in our decision by many friends and family. One day, Luke received a call from our pastor. He asked us if we would want to stand up in front of the church and tell everyone what was going on, and they would pray for us. Luke talked to me and we agreed to do it.

Sunday came and I was nervous. I didn't like knowing that everywhere we looked there were people who looked at us differently. But at the same time, I wanted people to care. We were often referred to as the pregnant/cancer couple.

We sat down in our usual seats near the back of the church. The worship songs began, and I bowed my head and let my tears go. Luke lovingly placed his arms around me. I quickly wiped my eyes as I did not want anyone to see my pain. I did not want to be pitied in any way. The music stopped and the pastor stepped up to the front of the church.

"Many of you are aware of the situation going on with Luke Bader, and I know you have been faithfully praying for him throughout his chemotherapy. Well, there is something else big that is going to take place very soon. I would like Luke and his wife, Michelle, to come up here please."

I struggled to get my large body through the row of people we were sitting with. Eyes wandered throughout the sanctuary as everyone looked to find us. I wondered what was going to be said. We were each given a stool to sit on.

"So, Luke, what is going to be happening next Thursday?" our pastor said as he handed a microphone to Luke.

"Well, I have a tumor in my right ankle, and I will be having a below-the-knee amputation done in order to remove it," Luke said confidently as though he had spoken in front of hundreds of people many times.

I looked out into the sea of faces and saw different emotions. Shock was the most prevalent. I saw tears welling up in eyes of people I had never even met. I wondered how they could care so much when they didn't even know us.

"Luke, you have a huge life-altering thing about to happen to you." The pastor then turned to the congregation. "I would like anyone who would like to support Luke and Michelle to come up here to the front and join me in prayer for them."

I heard the sounds of people getting out of their chairs. We were instantly surrounded by people in every direction. Hands were placed on us and tears fell from the eyes of many.

"Oh, God," the pastor began. "We thank you for this couple and the faith they have shown. They are an example to us all. Please be with Luke as the surgery is taking place. Guide the surgeons' hands. Please give strength to Luke and Michelle both. Give them the peace that only comes from you."

Tears flowed freely now from my hidden face. I was touched by his words and the support from the people around us, some that were strangers to me.

"We thank you for the many things you have given us, and we love you. Amen." The pastor concluded his prayer, and the people walked back to their seats.

"On top of all the physical things going on with Luke, there is the strain of him not being able work. This has taken a toll on their finances as well as the upcoming price of a prosthesis," the pastor said. I heard the words and thankfully realized the direction this was headed.

"I would like to do a love offering to help them out. If you would like to help support them, please give to them now as the offering plate is being passed around.

The music began to play, and we slowly walked back to our seats. I was once again touched by people's kindness. Just months before, my cousin Sherry set up an account in our name and sent letters to hundreds of people asking for financial help as well as prayers. We were amazed every day when we checked our bank account. There was always more money there. God provided for us in ways I never dreamed of.

As I watched the offering plate pass from person to person and saw countless checks and money being placed in it, I began to cry. This time the tears were thankful tears rather than painful tears.

You are awesome and indescribable, I prayed silently. *Thank you for these people, thank you for your love and peace and all the many things you have given us. Without you, we would be lost.*

God had answered our financial prayers. Now I wondered how he would answer the rest of the many prayers we had sent his way.

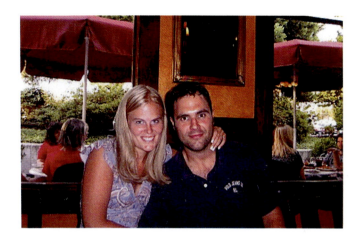

Our Rehearsal Dinner—August 21, 2003

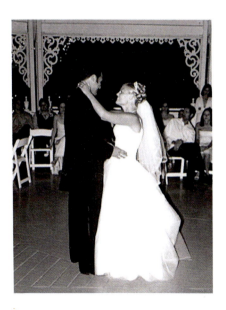

Our first dance at our wedding—August 22, 2003

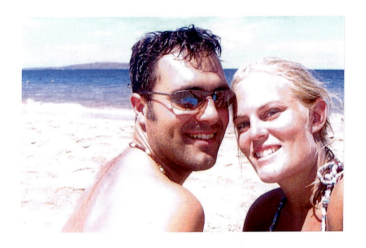

Our Honeymoon in Maui—August 2003

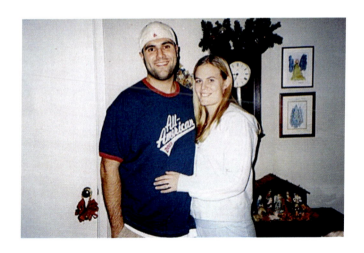

Our first Christmas, I was just pregnant
with Hayden—December 2003

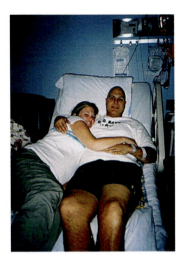

Luke in the hospital getting chemotherapy
while I was 6 month pregnant—April 2004

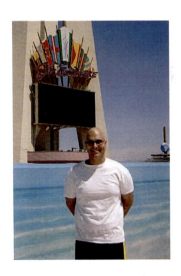

Our last vacation before Luke's amputation—April 2004

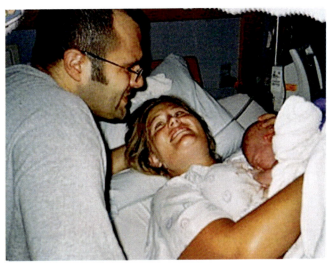

Luke looking at baby Hayden right
when he was born July 7, 2004

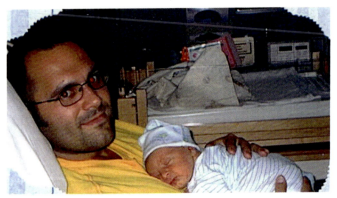

Luke holding newborn Hayden July 7, 2004

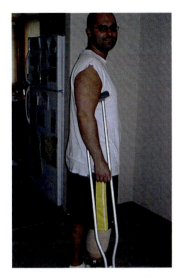

Luke learning to walk again—June 2004

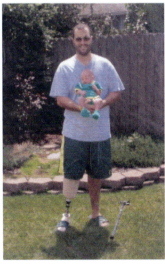

Luke holding Hayden while wearing
his first prosthesis July 2004

A Life-Changing Day

❦❧❦

eep, beep. I woke up abruptly to the sound of my screeching alarm and looked at the clock: 5:00 a.m. *Why am I getting up at this time?* My mind was fuzzy. I looked over at Luke and saw him sitting at the edge of the bed. Suddenly the reality of the day came over me as I realized what lay ahead.

It was the day of Luke's amputation. I had been dreading this day as well as looking forward to it to get rid of the cancer. I had cried many tears about this day, and I didn't know what to expect.

I knew Luke was nervous, scared, and anxious about this day. His head was bent down as though he was in silent prayer. I reached over and rubbed his back. As his feet hit the floor, I couldn't help thinking that would be the last time he would ever be able to place both feet on the ground and easily lift himself up. As he stood up and walked to the doorway, I looked at his legs. I could not picture him without one of them. I had tried to picture it many times in order to help myself prepare, but no matter what I did, the image would never come. Luke walked down the hall, and I felt myself beginning to weaken. Everything inside of me wanted to escape what was going on. *This can't be happening.*

I tried to keep the tears in and overcome my weakness with the appearance of strength. I recalled my conversation with Luke from the night before.

Luke looked down at his fettuccini Alfredo and pretended to be interested in eating it, but I knew he wasn't going to eat it. His mind was far away from our dinner of pasta.

"Baby," Luke said slowly as his eyes looked up to meet my own.

"Yes," I replied, reaching for his hand.

"You know I don't usually ask you for things, but I need you to do something for me tomorrow. I know everything will be emotional, but I really, really need you to be strong for me. Can you do that?" Luke said intently.

"Yes, it will be hard, but I will do my best," I said as I thought about how difficult the task would be.

Luke and I finished getting ready to go to the hospital in silence. We had been through packing for a hospital so many times that we could do it quickly and remember everything we could possibly need. In our then nine months of marriage, we had spent more time together in hospitals than hotels.

The drive to the hospital was equally as quiet as at home. I knew that Luke needed to deal with things in his way, and that was to be silent. I silently prayed for the upcoming day.

LORD, I give you this day, this day you have created. Please give Luke strength and courage to make it through this day. Please help the surgery to go well. Help the surgeon to do everything correctly and to get all the cancer out of his body. God, I don't know how I am going to be strong, but I know all things are possible through you. I feel like I could break down any second crying. Please help me to remain strong, at least until he is in surgery. Thanks, LORD.

I parked in the parking garage, and Luke and I began the walk into the hospital—the last time he would ever walk outside on his own two feet. There had been many last times that both Luke and I had thought of over the past few days: the last time he clipped his toenails, the last time he walked in our house, the last time he drove a car using his right leg only, and the last time he crossed his ankles.

Hand in hand, we walked slowly into the hospital. When we got to the waiting room, we were greeted by many friends and family who had come to show their support for Luke as well as me. Luke and I walked up to the counter where he was to check in. He was given many papers to sign and then we were told to wait, and they would let us know when there was a preop room ready for us to go into.

There was a unique stillness in our corner of the room. No one knew what to say. I looked around and quickly counted the people we knew. *Five, six, seven,* I continued counting. *Thirty-Five.* There were thirty-five people there for us. I looked at Luke's face and knew he was uncomfortable with all the attention. Luke did not like people to make a big deal out of things and would have preferred that only a few people were there. We waited for about two hours and were told we would have to wait longer still. I knew that Luke was anxious to get this surgery over with and start the recovery process. Friends and family continued to make small talk with us, and our pastor prayed over Luke. Finally, we were called back to the preop room. Only Luke and one other person were allowed, so naturally I went with him.

We began the walk down the long, sterile hallway, and I felt weakness trying to take over and form tears in my eyes. *I must be strong. I can hold out just a little longer. I promised Luke. I will do my best to be strong and not show my weakness until he is in surgery.* We were directed to a small room with a curtain for a door. Luke sat on the small hospital bed as I found a hard wooden chair to rest in. There were soon many nurses coming in and out of the room taking blood pressure, temperatures, etc. I looked at Luke's two legs at the edge of the bed. I could see the lump on his right leg. *We are getting rid of you today, cancer! I will not think of it as Luke losing a leg, but Luke losing the cancer!*

After a while, the room became quieter and the people coming in and going out became fewer. Soon Luke and I were left alone.

"Come here, baby," Luke said as he scooted over on the tiny hospital bed and patted the space next to him. We had shared hospital beds many times before, so it did not surprise me when he wanted me to join him on this day. I placed one leg up and tried to balance the rest of my body to fit on the bed. I barely fit. I lay my head upon Luke's chest and listened to the sound of his steady, calming heartbeat. I closed my eyes and knew that everything was going to be okay. I pictured Luke and I on a boat; the waves crashed at us from every side, but our sturdy boat kept us safe. I knew that someday the waves would calm, and the stillness of the sea would overpower the memories of the crashing waves, and life would be better again.

Luke and I lay in silence for many minutes. We did not have to speak to know what was going on in each other's minds. It was such a foreign thought to know that in just a little while, my husband's life would be dramatically different. Not just my husband's life but mine as well. We were one in every sense of the word. When he was hurting, so was I.

"Knock, knock," I heard a voice say. I looked up to see Luke's mom entering the room.

"Hi," Luke replied.

"I just want to make sure they get the right one," Luke's mom said as she pulled a pen out from her purse. She proceeded to take the pen and write on his left leg "NOT THIS ONE!".

"That's a good idea," I said, laughing. It felt good to laugh. Laughter had not happened very much lately in our house, and I missed it. I missed the sound of Luke's laugh and the way his eyes brightened with every bubble of laughter he produced. I prayed that laughter would once again be a part of our lives soon.

"Well, I better get going. I love you," Luke's mom said as she leaned over and kissed his forehead. I could see that she was holding back tears that were fighting their way to the brim of her eyes. She turned around and left quickly before the tears could fall. Soon a nurse entered the tiny room.

"It is time to get your epidural started," he said as he moved things around on his medical tray.

I looked at Luke. He knew how much I hated needles and how much I was already scared of the epidural I would have in a few months.

"I think I will wait outside," I said as I kissed Luke lightly on the cheek.

I walked up and down the hall, trying to calm myself. I looked at my watch. Ten minutes had passed, I knew they had to be done by now. I walked back down the hall and stood outside the room. The curtain moved and I was able to see a tiny sliver of Luke. I saw his bare back bent over and the nurse trying to place what I assumed was the needle in his back. I quickly turned away and tried to keep myself together. I did not like to see anything that caused pain, and it looked like Luke was probably in pain. I paced up and down the hall a few times and I saw the curtain to Luke's room open. I quickly made my way back to the room.

Luke was lying on the bed with his eyes closed and a look of pain on his face.

"How are you?" I asked.

"It really hurt. I don't think that guy knew what he was doing. He had to do it over and over, I think five times!" Luke said.

"I am so sorry," I said as I sat down beside him. My stomach was tense and I was tired of waiting. I wanted to get the surgery over with. Within a few minutes, a nurse came in.

"Well, it is time to go. We will give you your anesthesia in another room, so you will be out for the surgery," she said.

"Yes. Please make sure that the drugs are really strong. I want to be out. I do not want to wake up during the surgery," Luke said directly.

"Yes, of course. We will make sure you do not wake up during the surgery," the nurse replied.

The curtain to Luke's room was now wide open and things were moved to the side as they prepared to wheel Luke's bed down the hall. Suddenly I felt as though I was in a dream. Everything was fuzzy. I bent down over Luke and kissed him.

"I love you," I said softly.

He looked up at me. "I love you too," Luke said as they began to roll his bed away. I watched his body move farther away from me. I stared at his leg one last time and wondered what he would be like without it. When I could no longer see Luke, all the strength that had been holding back my tears dissipated under the weight of my emotions. I leaned against the wall and felt my body slowly sliding to the floor. I felt the cold, hard floor beneath me. I buried my face in my hands and began to sob. I could hardly catch my breath. My chest rose and fell quickly, and the saltiness of my tears flowed into my mouth. I did not look up. I couldn't hear anyone, I couldn't feel anything but intense pain in my heart. *God, why? Why is this happening to him? I can't handle to see this happening to him!* I prayed. I felt a hand on my shoulder.

"Sweetie, do you have anyone here with you?" I looked up to the kind face of a nurse.

"Yes," I said as I wiped my eyes with my shirt.

I stood up and made my way to the doors that led to the waiting room. I did not want to see anyone. No one could comfort the kind of pain I was feeling. Instead of going to the waiting room, I walked to the bathroom. I found an empty stall, sat down, closed the door, and let the tears cascade down my face once again.

"Please God, please God, please God," I said the words aloud as I rocked back and forth. I could not pray any other words. God knew the intense feelings and the prayers I felt from deep inside. I looked at my bracelet which was made up of photos of Luke and I. I rubbed the pictures over and over. "Please God, please God, please God." Those were the only words that would come out of my lips. I didn't know how else to pray. I had never felt so in need of comfort. *Please God*—those two words came from a longing from the depths of my being to be held and comforted by my Savior.

I continued crying until I felt strong enough to go out and face other people. I walked out of the stall and looked in the mirror. My eyes were puffy, my cheeks were red, and I had mascara all around my eyes. I wiped my face and tried to make myself look a little less upset. *I don't really care what I look like right now.*

I rubbed my belly and said, "Don't worry, Hayden. Daddy is going to be okay." Talking to Hayden made me feel better. I felt like I was ready to face other people. I opened the door and walked to the waiting room. I was immediately engulfed in the arms of many caring people. I was comforted by their love and touched by their emotions.

"So, he is in surgery now?" my mom asked.

"Well, he was going to the room where they put him out, and then he will go to surgery," I said. I looked down at the pager I had been given. I was told that when Luke was in recovery I would be paged and they would let me know how everything went. I didn't know how I was going to wait the long six hours until they predicted he would be done. I sat down next to the others in the waiting room and tried to pass the time. I looked at magazines, but somehow the "Top Ten Ways to Lose Weight" didn't seem to keep my interest. I just kept imagining what my sweet Luke was going through. I pictured him lying on the operating table as the surgeon began to cut his leg. *Awh*, it was too awful I just couldn't think about it anymore. I decided I would go for a walk to help pass more time. I was getting rather large as I neared my eighth month of pregnancy, and I knew walking would be good for me.

As I began down the hall, I heard my cell phone ring.

"Hello," I said.

"Hey, it's Amanda. I was just wondering how everything was going."

I was happy that she remembered even from Canada to call and check in on me. Amanda had always been such a good friend to me since we met when we were fourteen years old. It was comforting to hear her voice. I proceeded to explain the events of the morning and told her I would call her again when Luke was out of surgery.

I hung up the phone and continued walking down the hall. I was still feeling sick to my stomach yet a bit hungry. Although I didn't feel like eating, I knew that Hayden needed me to. I went back to the waiting room and noticed that several people had left. There really wasn't much good in them waiting around all day anyways. There were still several people left to support me and be there for Luke when he awoke. My family and Luke's family remained.

I walked over to the corner where everyone was sitting. Well, my dad was sleeping on a couch but everyone else were sitting quietly reading or pretending to read.

"Does anyone want to get some lunch?" I said.

"That sounds good," my mom said as she stood up. My sisters-in-law Amy and Jessica, and Luke's mom and sister Trudee got up too. We walked down to the cafeteria. I decided on a chicken-and-cheese sandwich. I ordered and sat down at a booth. *How can I eat right now? This is wrong! I feel so guilty eating while Luke's leg is being cut off. How can I do this?* I took a small bite off my sandwich; it did not taste good to me. I pushed it around on my plate absentmindedly and hoped that no one would notice.

"Aren't you going to eat?" my mom asked.

"I don't feel like it," I said.

"Well, you need to eat," my mom said in a very motherly tone.

I took one more bite and decided I couldn't eat anymore. When we were done, we walked back to the waiting room and tried to pass the time once again. The hours seemed to drag on forever. Six hours had passed and my pager had not gone off. I began to get a little nervous. *What if something went wrong? That would be too much for me to handle, and God promised me he won't give me more than I can handle.*

Dinnertime came and went, and I suddenly felt a buzz at my hip where I had the pager attached. Luke was out of surgery! I rushed to the counter and told them I had been paged. They told me the surgeon would be with me shortly.

I tried to wait as patiently as I could, but my patience had already been used up over the entire day. I looked up from where I was sitting and saw the surgeon—a woman dressed in scrubs, in her mid-thirties—walking toward me. She looked directly at me.

"Hi. It went really well."

I felt relief spread throughout my entire body.

"We had to keep him in recovery for longer than expected because he was out for a long time. We got the tumor out, and I had room to leave a large margin of space from where the tumor was to where the leg was cut. Luke is doing well and is now in his own room on the tenth floor. I will be back tomorrow to check on him," she said.

I wanted to find the elevator and see Luke as soon as possible. She continued talking for a few more minutes, but all I could think of was seeing Luke's face. I was given his room number and we went toward his room. We got off the elevator and got closer to his room. Luke's mom was the only one with me.

"You go ahead," she said to me. I appreciated that she would give Luke and I a few minutes alone. As I continued down the hall, I was overcome with emotions. Since the first date Luke and I had been on, I had never felt so nervous to see him. *What would he be like? Would he be angry? Upset? Scared? Tired?* I was unsure of how I would react to seeing him with part of his leg gone. *Would it be bloody?* I had a hard time with blood, but I was ready to face anything to see my Luke. He would still be my same wonderful, caring husband, and I couldn't wait to lay eyes on him again.

I entered the doorway to Luke's room. I saw him sitting up in his bed. His body was covered in a pale-blue blanket. I could see that underneath the blanket was his left leg and foot, and the blanket lay flat below his right knee where his leg should have been. His face looked peaceful.

"Hey, baby," I said as I walked to the side of his bed. "How are you doing?"

Luke looked up at me with a smile. "Much better than I thought I would be. It was so scary, I woke up in the recovery room and I couldn't move. I tried to move my arms and legs, but nothing would work. I was so scared that something had gone wrong in the surgery and I would be paralyzed forever. I called the nurse over and asked her what was happening, and she told me that it was the anesthesia, and it would soon wear off. It wasn't long until I could start to move again. I thanked God. It really put things into perspective for me. It made me thankful that I only lost a leg compared to being paralyzed forever."

With each word that Luke said, I was amazed at his calmness and peace. It was truly a miracle from God. There was no other way to explain the peace that came from deep inside his soul. I was in awe of my husband. He was so strong, even after his leg had been taken.

"Do you want to see it?" Luke said as he studied my face for a reaction. "It's not bloody or anything." Luke reached for the blanket covering his legs.

"Okay," I replied, nervous as to what I would see.

He pulled the blanket off and revealed a white plaster cast. The cast extended about two inches below his knee where it ended. I let out a sigh of relief. It was not such a scary sight.

"You are right, it isn't bloody. Does it hurt?" I bent down and examined the cast.

"Well, I can't feel either of my legs very well right now, but it is starting to throb a little."

"What is this?" I asked as I looked at a small blood-filled tube at the end of his cast. Even as I looked at it, I was surprised that I did not become weak from the sight of blood.

"That is for the blood that is still draining out of my leg," Luke replied.

"I am so proud of you, Luke. You are being so strong," I said as I kissed Luke gently. "I need to go get your mom, she is waiting outside."

Luke's mom walked in and gave Luke a hug. They talked for awhile and then she said she would leave and let him rest. I could tell by the way Luke's face was tensing up that he was beginning to feel more pain.

"It hurts."

I knew it must be bad because Luke never complained about pain. "Did you get pain medicine?" I asked.

"Yes, and there is some going through my epidural, but the pain is getting worse!"

I closed my eyes and prayed that somehow we would make it through another pain-filled night—a night that was to be the worst night of our lives.

Where Are You, God?

The pain grew more intense by the second. The look of peace had now faded from Luke's face and was replaced by anguish. "I think I will call a nurse in to see if they can give me more pain medicine."

"That's a good idea," I said, desperately wanting to be able to help in some way.

Luke pushed the button that called the nurse to come in.

Within a few minutes, a nurse was in the room. "How can I help you?"

Luke looked at her, trying to remain calm. "My leg really hurts, and I need some more medication."

"Okay, just a minute. Let me see what I can do." She said it in a way that told me she didn't really care about Luke's pain. She returned within a few minutes. "Well, it looks like we have given you all the pain meds we are authorized to give you. Tomorrow, when we talk to the doctor, we may be able to get you some more."

I looked at Luke and saw his eyes squeezed together and his lips tight. I knew he was angry and in immense pain.

The nurse turned to walk out the door, and I had the urge to run after her and tackle her to the floor. How could she be so cold and uncaring? She has no heart. She could have said it a little nicer. I would like to cut off her skinny little legs! My thoughts became angrier each time I looked at my husband and saw what was happening to him. There was no relief for his pain, nothing I could do to stop the hurt. He was suffering, and all I could do was sit beside him and watch helplessly as he endured the worst pain of his life.

Deeper into the night, Luke still was not able to sleep. He called for the nurse again. "Yes, I was wondering if you could check and see if my epidural is still working? It feels like it might be off," Luke said desperately.

The nurse proceeded to check the little tube hooked up to his epidural.

"No, it looks like it is hooked up and still going," she said, and she walked out the door.

Luke's face was tensed up in pain as it had been all night. I saw tears beginning to roll down his cheeks. As I watched him, my own tears began to fall as well. I reached out for his hand. Together, we cried in silence.

"I am going to pray for you, Luke." I said.

"God, we really need you now. Please, please take away the pain. Luke is hurting so much. Please, please, please." I wiped away my ever-flowing tears. "Luke can't get any more medicine and there is nothing we can do. Can you hear us? Are you there God!" I said in a loud voice.

Luke was crying hard now, the hardest I had ever seen him cry over pain. "Please, please, please," Luke cried desperately as his voice wavered with every syllable he spoke. My heart had never been broken as much as it was at that moment. There was nothing worse than watching the man I love cry out in pain for help. All the physical strength had been taken from Luke and was replaced by pain so deep and intense that he could not even describe it to me.

Luke's cries were so painful and unnatural. He clenched his pillow in his fists and let out the most excruciating sound I had ever heard.

God, please! Can't you hear him! Can't you help him? Why must he suffer? Why must he go through this? Do something, please! Do you hear us? Can you hear our prayers? I cried out silently to God.

Be still and know that I am God. The words came into my head suddenly.

How can I be still? I thought. *I know you are God, but how can I be still and do nothing?*

The words spoke to me again, and I began to feel a little bit more at peace. Luke's cries were beginning to lessen, and I decided that maybe God was right after all. Instead of getting angry, I should try to have peace and be still.

I looked over at Luke. His eyes were wide open.

"Do you think you can sleep?" I asked.

"No, but I want you to try." Luke replied.

"Okay," I said as I lay down on my small fold-out bed. I found my CD player and put on my headphones. Soon the soothing sounds of Norah Jones surrounded me. My tears continued to flow as I tried to lose myself in the music. The music helped me to relax and I finally drifted off to sleep, at least for a few hours.

I awoke to the sun shining through the curtains. I looked at Luke. He was sitting up in his bed. A look of pain still occupied his face.

"How did you sleep?" I asked, hopeful for his rest.

"I didn't," he replied quickly.

"Baby, I am sorry. How is the pain?" I asked.

"Still pretty bad, but they came in a few minutes ago and said that my surgeon will be coming to check on me, so hopefully then I can get some better meds."

I hoped that the surgeon would be able to get Luke some more pain medication; I did not want him to suffer anymore.

The morning was filled with many people coming to check on Luke. First there was a physical therapist. She wanted to see if Luke was able to get out of bed yet. They tried but he was just in too much pain. He was still unable to feel either of his legs, so this made it difficult to try moving around. Next, a nurse came in to get Luke's breakfast order. Though Luke was in pain, he still had his usual appetite which made me happy. Finally, after hours of waiting, the surgeon came in.

"Hi, Luke, how are you doing?" the surgeon said as she walked through the doorway.

"I am in a lot of pain," Luke quickly replied.

"I will make sure you get more pain medication. You should be in some pain, but not intolerable pain. What's your pain level right now?" she asked.

I knew that she was referring to the chart on the wall that showed happy and sad faces next to different numbers, ten being the worst and having the saddest face. Luke and I had often made fun of the chart and referred to it often jokingly. Usually, when asked during chemo, he would say his pain level was around a four.

"Eleven," Luke replied knowing that was off the chart pain. "And it has been like that since last night."

"And you weren't given anything? You should have been given medicine last night. There is no reason for you to be in that much pain," she said with just enough emotion in her voice to make me wonder if she was a doctor that had emotions and really cared about Luke's well being. So far, I had not seen many doctors of that kind. "I will make sure that is taken care of immediately," she continued as she walked out the door. She soon returned and approached Luke's cast.

"It looks like it is draining properly," she said as she inspected the blood-draining tube. "Make sure you are keeping it elevated. Can you lift it for me?"

I could see Luke straining to lift, but nothing happened. "I still can't feel either of my legs. Is that normal?" Luke asked, concerned.

"Yes, you will probably regain feeling today," she said.

As I watched them talk, I couldn't help feeling proud of my husband. Despite his pain and current situation, he still remained positive. He truly was the best man in the world. What other person could go through all that he did and still remain so positive?

Luke was soon given more pain medication, and I could see a small amount of relief come over him. I knew he was still in pain but less than before.

The day passed slowly as I watched my husband in pain. It was night again and Luke had still not slept. I looked over at him on the small hospital bed. I peered once again at his altered leg. I was surprised how I was already getting used to seeing him in the cast. I knew that it may be different when the cast was off and I was able to see his actual leg for the first time. He was still the same man I had married just nine months earlier. Many hard things had happened to him and instead of defeating him, they made him stronger. The man I sat with in the hospital was my same husband, yet stronger in spirit. He had become amazingly close to God and showed me what it really meant to trust God no matter what.

Another sleepless night was upon us, and I prayed once again that Luke might have some relief from his pain. I looked over at Luke and wondered if I would be able to sleep.

"Luke," I said quietly as I watched him lying on his bed with eyes shut.

"Ya," Luke replied, his eye fluttering open.

"I really am praying that you can sleep tonight. You really need it. How is your pain? Do you think you can sleep?" I asked, hopeful.

"My pain is better and I am super tired, so of course I am hoping that I can sleep," replied Luke.

"Well, goodnight, my love. Let's both try to get some rest," I said and kissed him on the cheek then tried to lie down on my pull-out bed. My seven-months-pregnant body was having a really difficult time cramming into the tiny bed. *Ouch, this is really tiny and squished!* Then I told myself, *Michelle, don't be so selfish! Look at what Luke is suffering through!*

I closed my eyes, and soon the exhaustion of the past few days took over, and I fell asleep. I fell into a deep sleep, the kind of sleep that makes you feel as if you are lost in another world. I do not remember dreaming, but my body was relaxed and peaceful. I awoke early to the sounds of a nurse taking Luke's breakfast order. As usual, he ordered many things for breakfast, which is his favorite meal. The day was once again occupied by the visits of many specialists. Today, Luke was going to try using a walker to walk down the hall.

"Hey. Luke. How are you doing today?" came the words from the physical therapist who entered the room.

"All right. I can feel my legs again. I would like to try to get out of bed today," Luke said.

"Well, we can try to make that happen today," the therapist replied.

Luke brought his legs around to the side of the small hospital bed. His left foot touched the floor while his other leg hung just below his knee. There were a series of cords and wires that had to be moved in order for Luke to get up. The therapist placed the walker in front of him.

"I want you to start by putting all of your weight on you arms and your left leg," he said as Luke stood up on his only foot and placed his hands on the metal rims of the walker.

"Great. Now lets try and take a step."

Luke proceeded to use his arms to move the walker as his left foot left the floor and came directly behind his arms. I placed my hand on his back and whispered, "Good job, baby." I knew that not only was this physically difficult but even more emotionally hard for him. This was very humbling for him. Who would have ever thought Luke, the baseball star and athlete, would ever have to learn to walk again with one foot?

"Let's try walking down the hall," said the therapist.

Luke proceeded to take one step after another. His face was tight in concentration, and I could see that this was extremely difficult for him to do. He would never complain about his exhaustion but would continue to push through it. It was Luke's first time to be out of bed since his surgery.

I held my breath as I watched Luke trying to move his weak body. I did not want him to be discouraged if he could not do it. Slowly, he made it to the doorway and proceeded out into the hallway. I could see sweat forming on his forehead. He used the walker and made it to the end of the hallway. I was so proud of him. I could only imagine how difficult each step was for him. After a few minutes, he made his return to the room and I helped him back into bed.

"You did so good. I am proud of you!" I said to Luke, stroking his sweaty face with my hand.

"Thank you, sweetie," Luke said as he lay back on his pillow and closed his eyes.

Luke rested for a few more hours and decided that he wanted to get out of the room again. We had a wheelchair brought into the room, and I helped him get in it. I got behind him and tried to push him down the hall. This was a difficult task because I was seven months pregnant. As we walked down the hall, I thought to myself that we must look like quite a pair. We made it to the elevator and began our descent to the third floor. Luke wanted to go outside. I wheeled him through the cafeteria and was aware of people looking at us out of curiosity. I don't care what they think! They have no idea what we are going through!

We approached the glass doors that led to the courtyard, and I tried to figure out how I was going to open the door and push Luke through at the same time. I decided to place my back against the door and push with all of my strength while pulling Luke's chair with me. I looked around. *Why doesn't anyone offer to help me? How can people be so self-absorbed?* After a short struggle, we were outside.

The fresh, crisp air felt good on my face. The tree leaves rustled from the small breeze. I brought Luke over near a bench and I sat down next to him.

"It is nice to be outside," Luke said as he breathed in deeply.

"Yes, I am glad they let us go somewhere by ourselves," I said.

We sat outside for a few minutes in silence. I never ever imagined this would be our life. *It's just not fair!* I thought as I looked at my husband. He looked so pale, his bald head a reminder of chemotherapy. His absence of a lower leg and foot was still a shock to my eyes. This must be some kind of nightmare I am going to wake up from any second. *How in the world could this be real?* I thought bitterly. No mater how much I had prepared myself for the surgery, it was still very hard for me emotionally.

After a few moments in the fresh air, we decided it was time to go back upstairs to Luke's room so he could rest. I wheeled him again through the cafeteria, paying no attention to the other people. We returned to Luke's room and I helped him get from his wheelchair to the bed. I could see pain spreading across his face, and I was glad that I had brought him back to rest more.

As I watched Luke close his eyes, I closed my eyes and tried to rest as well. The sunlight felt warm on my face. The gentle heat made me feel more peaceful. *Why am I being so bitter? This is God's plan for my life, and when things are tough, I need to remember that. Who knows how God is going to use all of this in someone's life? Seriously, Michelle, you have got to stop getting angry and rest in the peace that God is in control*, I told myself. I decided once again that I was going to try my best to have a good attitude and not let bitterness continue to dwell in me.

Later that day, we had some visitors. Luke's parents walked through the room. His mom walked right up to him with a smile. His dad was close behind. I could see him looking at the cast on Luke's leg that ended a few inches below his knee. His face began to tense, as Luke's often did, and his eyes swelled with tears. He began to sniffle and he covered his face.

"Oh, Son," he said through a strained voice. "I would take your place if I could," he said as he began to cry harder. He turned around and walked out the door. I looked at Luke and there were tears in his eyes. I began to cry once again. I did not fully understand why Luke's dad was taking it so hard. I was not yet a parent and did not know how it would feel to see your son in pain.

After a few minutes, we had all gained our composure, and Luke's dad returned.

The next few days, we had many friends and family visiting, and after five long nights, we were ready to go home. Even before Luke's surgery, we had prepared our house for his return. We had a wheelchair, crutches, and a walker ready for him to use.

It was the day we were to leave, and I was very excited to return home. I busily packed up all of our things and waited for Luke to be discharged from the hospital.

"All right, it looks like you guys are free to go," a nurse said to me as she handed me a bunch of papers. Both my mom and Luke's mom were helping us. They helped us gather all of our things and we began our decent to the main hospital floor. I pushed Luke to the main entrance.

"I will get your car," my mom said. I handed her the keys.

We waited a few minutes and soon saw our bright-yellow bug pull up. I opened the passenger side and helped Luke into the seat. It was a small car and it was difficult at first for Luke to even get in the car. After much struggling, Luke found a way to sit down. I piled pillows under Luke's leg.

"How does that feel, baby?" I said.

"It's okay, but I think I need another pillow to elevate it more."

I rummaged through the things in our car until I found another pillow. I placed it under his cast.

"How is that?"

"Better."

I closed his door.

"Do you think you need some help at home?" my mom asked.

"I think we will be okay. Luke would rather do it alone. We have all the things we need. I will call if I need anything," I said.

"Okay, love you." my mom said.

"Love you too." I walked to my side of the car and got in next to Luke. We began the journey home. As we approached the freeway, I noticed all the cars ahead of us.

"Traffic," I said intently. *I hate traffic, but I know I need to remain calm for Luke's sake,* I thought to myself. We inched onto the freeway. I glanced over at Luke. His eyes were closed and his face was tight.

"What is it, baby?" I asked.

"My leg is really throbbing. Let's just get home as soon as possible."

It took us well over an hour to make the usual half-hour trip home. We pulled into the garage. I gave the crutches to Luke and he slowly began to crutch his way to the house. He went straight for our bedroom. He made it to the bed and collapsed on it. His face showed pure exhaustion and pain. I knew I needed to let him rest.

"What can I get you?" I asked.

"Just some water for now," Luke said. I grabbed two cups and filled them up with water. I knew that Luke liked to keep two glasses of water next to him.

After I filled up the water, I walked around the house. *What should I do now? I want to help him, but there is nothing I can do.* I thought. *Well, I guess there is one thing that I can do. I can pray. Yes, that is what I will do. Though I don't know the outcome of my prayers or why God chooses to answer things differently than I want, I can still pray.* I sat down on the couch and closed my weary eyes.

Oh, God, I come to you today and I am weak. I do not know what to do. I do not understand why Luke has to go through this. Please help me to know what to do to be the supportive wife that he needs. God, I am sorry for the times I have complained about everything. You do have a plan. You created me for this. I am going to do everything I can to help Luke and not be bitter. Please, LORD, please take away Luke's pain. Help him to be able to rest—to rest both physically and emotionally. I know this has been incredibly hard on him, harder than most people will ever know. Help me to show him every day how much I love him and how proud I am of him. I want him to know that. Thank you for being my strength and my rock. I love you. Amen.

I lifted my head and wiped my tears. I was ready to be what Luke needed me to be. I was ready for the future, I was ready for the unknown, and I was most definitely ready for the journey of Luke's recovery to begin.

The Healing Journey

*T*he first days at home were difficult ones. Luke was not used to asking me for things, and he hated depending on someone else. He was learning how to get around our house using different devices. He used crutches, a wheelchair, and a walker. Most of his time was spent on the recliner in the front room. This day was no different. I walked around the corner and saw Luke reclined in his chair.

"Hey, baby, how are you doing?" I asked.

"Okay," he replied as his leg suddenly jerked.

"Are you having phantom pains?" I said thinking of how I hated the phantom pains. Luke had explained phantom pains to me several times. They are very common with amputees. There are still nerves where the limb has been removed and the brain still sends signals that often have pain attached to them.

"Yes, this time it is the electric-shock pain." Luke's face was tensed in pain. Luke had told me before that there were several different pains he experienced. In addition to the shock, there was a burning feeling like his foot was on fire, a sensation that a nail was piercing his foot, and a feeling of his foot being crushed into pieces.

My heart went out to him as I watched the way his face tightened every time there was another phantom pain. *I wish there was something that I could do. I hate seeing him in so much pain! Why does he have to go through all of this? I still don't understand. I will trust God that there is some kind of plan for all of this pain.*

"Can I get you anything?" I asked, knowing that he would not want to ask me.

"Ya, can you get me some water?" Luke said.

I watched the water cascade from the faucet and splash into the blue plastic cup. I loved helping Luke but was having a hard time as my energy was decreasing daily. I was nearing the end of my third trimester and Hayden would soon be born. *I wish I wasn't so tired and I could help more!* I thought as I returned to the front room and handed the water to Luke.

"Thank you," Luke said quietly.

I leaned over and kissed him softly on the forehead. I looked at my watch; it was almost time for me to leave for work. I was nervous leaving as I had not left Luke since his surgery. I was thankful for our friends and family. Luke's mom was coming over and I knew she would take good care of him and get him everything he needed.

We had already been blessed by our friends. Every night since we had been home, there had been a hot meal delivered to us. All the wonderful people from work also sent us many gift certificates to restaurants where I could get takeout. We were amazed at the ways God provided for us. There was not a day that went by that we did not feel his peace.

Ding-Dong. The doorbell interrupted my thoughts. I waddled to the door and slowly opened it.

"Hi," I greeted Luke's Mom.

"Hi, how is he doing?" she said.

"He is having a lot of phantom pains today. I am really glad you are here to help. I feel bad leaving, but I really can't miss any more days. There are only a few weeks of school left and I really need to be there."

"I am glad that I can help. Don't worry, I will take care of him," she said as if she could read the worry on my face.

"Bye, baby," I said as I kissed Luke good-bye and headed to my car. I knew I would be facing another day of awkward questions from people who didn't know what to say. I wanted to go back in the house, crawl into bed, and never face another person again.

Suddenly, the sweet and curious faces of my kindergarteners came into my head. *They need me today. They are counting on me. I have to face life even if it is just for them. I feel bad that they have already had substitute teachers so many times.*

God had placed me in this position for a reason. He knew I was strong enough to deal with everything placed before me. *I can do all these things! I can be a support to Luke through all this, be a great teacher, get my master's degree, and be eight months pregnant all during my first year of marriage. Wow, God must think I am pretty tough to endure all this. He knows I will not give up and let the circumstances drown me. I will persevere. Just think of how strong Luke and I will be after all that we have been through!* I was suddenly energized and motivated to face the day as I realized that God had given me strength and peace beyond what I ever imagined possible. I whispered a prayer of thanks to my peace-giver.

"Thank you, Jesus. Thank you for suddenly motivating me to persevere through these days, the hardest days of my life. Honestly, God, there are days when I feel really sorry for myself and I don't want to talk to anyone. Thank you for helping me realize that you have a plan for me, and that plan does not involve giving up and feeling sorry for myself. You have picked me up and filled me with your holy peace and divine strength. One single tear slowly slid down my face. *God, I feel closer to you than I ever have in my life. I don't know what I would do if I didn't have you. Where would my strength come from? I certainly wouldn't have enough strength on my own to get through even one day. God, I want to remember this day when I see others hurting. I want to be able to share how much you have done for me. I want others who are hurting to feel this same peace and strength that you have given to me. God, help me to be your vessel of hope, of peace, and of strength.*

I felt better after praying. I walked into my colorful classroom and knew that in fact, God had given me the strength to get through not only that day but many, many more. I did survive the day and returned home to my amazing husband.

He was asleep when I walked into our room. I watched him breathe, and peace flowed through my body. *The cancer is gone! I know his leg is gone, but the up side is, so is the cancer!* Luke's chest rose and fell with a steady and consistent pace as I continued to study his face. His hair was starting to grow back. I could see fine lashes beginning to form on his eyelids. The hair regrowth encouraged me. It was a sign of healing, a beam of hope for a new future.

The days continued in pretty much the same manner. I would leave for work and Luke's mom would come over to help take care of him. It was so nice to know that someone was at home with Luke. I also enjoyed coming home to a sparkling clean house. She would clean when Luke was resting. I was glad she was, because cleaning was not on the list of my priorities for the time being.

After two weeks, the first big step in Luke's recovery happened. The first cast was removed! He went through two more casts until finally they were all removed. I came home after work to see Luke's leg for the first time. I walked into our bedroom to see Luke sitting up in the bed.

"Hi," I said as I kissed him gently. "How did it go today?" I glanced at the sheet covering his leg.

"Pretty good. Do you want to see my leg without the cast?" he asked.

"Ya, I think I can handle it," I said, unsure of what I was about to see.

Luke slowly pulled the sheet back. I saw his newly altered leg. Everything looked as it used to until about two inches below his knee. At the end of his leg, there were some staples. I could see blood had formed near the edges of the staples.

"Does it hurt?" I asked.

"Not that bad right now. The doctor said my staples are healing very well and in a few weeks I can start getting fit for my prosthesis," Luke said with some excitement in his voice. I knew that he was looking forward to having a prosthesis and regaining his independence.

"That is great news, baby! I am excited for you," I said.

I looked at Luke and realized that he was in an unusually energetic mood. I guess the promise of independence had made him joyful.

"Michelle, I know it has been driving you crazy that we have not been out of the house together in weeks. I was wondering if you would want to take me for a drive."

"Yes, yes, yes!" I exclaimed as I leaned over to kiss him. Luke knew me so well. He knew how hard it was for me not to be able to go anywhere with him. *My husband is so sweet and thoughtful even through his pain. I am truly blessed to have him for my husband!* I thought while preparing to leave. I gathered up three pillows, as I knew Luke would need some padding to put his sensitive leg on.

Click, click, click. I heard the sound of Luke's crutches going down the hall. He was getting pretty good at using those. I did feel bad for him when he told me that using them created sores under his arms.

"Are you ready to go?" I said as I opened the door to the garage. I looked around to make sure there was nothing that would block Luke's path. I was now aware of things that might pose a problem for him to maneuver around. I always did my best to remove those things from his way.

"Yes, I am coming," he said and crutched his way to the garage. I opened the bright-yellow car door for him. Once again, I was aware that a new beetle was a difficult car for our present situation. He seated himself in the car and dropped his crutches to the ground. *I guess he won't be needing those since we are not getting out anywhere,* I thought to myself as I sat down behind the wheel. I suddenly realized I had no idea where we were going. I had been so excited about getting out of the house with Luke that I didn't even think about it.

"Where do you want to go?" I asked.

"I am not sure. Just a nice drive, somewhere pretty." Luke replied.

"How about Hockinson? We could go look at the big houses," I said. Hockinson was the community where I worked. It was known for its beautiful countryside and nice homes.

"Sure. I don't care where we go, it will just be nice to be out with you." Luke smiled at me. We began the picturesque drive to Hockinson. As we entered the wide open beauty, I realized how thankful I was for the healing that was taking place inside of Luke. A year prior, a drive with Luke would not have meant so much. Now, the simple beauty of life had the power to take my breath away.

As we drove farther up, I could see the beauty of Mount St. Helens to my left. The sun shone down on it and the sky was crystal clear. *What a perfect day for this!* I thought to myself. We drove around for a while and I looked over at Luke. I could tell that something was wrong.

"What is it, baby?" I asked.

"I am starting to be in pain. Can we go home now?" he said.

"Of course," I said as I turned the car around to head toward home. I knew that he had probably been hurting for a while and didn't want to say anything to me because he knew how much I was enjoying being out with him. That's the kind of man I married. He always put me first and sacrificed his own well being in order to make me happy. *I couldn't have married a better man! Even though these are the hardest times in my life, I have never regretted marrying Luke for a second. Even if I knew all of this was ahead of us on our wedding day, I would still have gladly married my Luke. What God has joined together, let no man or cancer destroy!*

We returned home and Luke lay down to rest. It felt so good to be able to be with Luke somewhere other than our house. I could only imagine the cabin fever he must be feeling; not only from being stuck in the house but from not being able to move around the way he was used to. I had often tried to imagine what it would be like to look down and not see my foot. I imagined how it must feel to have to grab the crutches to get up and go even a short distance.

Every day, my respect for my husband grew more and more as I watched the many hard things that he had to endure. *I wonder if things will ever get better,* I thought to myself. *Well, they already have improved so much, I just know they will!* I tried my best to keep a positive attitude even though things were very difficult.

After three casts, Luke was finally ready to be fit for his prosthesis.

The day of Luke's appointment soon approached. I wanted to take him to his appointment but he said that I didn't need to take any more days off from work. His mom took him to the appointment.

The process for getting prosthesis is a lengthy one. The first time that Luke went to his appointment, they measured his leg to see what size to make his prosthesis. Weeks later, he went back and he was finally given his leg. I came home to him standing in front of the mirror.

"Wow, Luke!" I said as I looked at my husband. He was standing in front of our full-length mirror with crutches under his arms. I felt warm tears filling my eyes. *It sure is good to see him stand! It has been a long time since I have seen that! What a miracle. We do have a happier future in store!*

He looked good standing on two legs. His prosthesis was not complete yet, and its bottom was made of a metal pole.

"What do you think?" Luke said to me with a smile on his face.

"I think it looks great! Can you show me how you can walk?"

"Ya. My doctor said that it helps to look at a mirror while practicing."

Luke crutched his way down the hall and turned to face the mirror. Slowly, he placed his new right leg in front of him. His left leg followed, and he used his crutches for balance. He continued all the way down the hall until he reached the mirror.

"Great job! I am so proud of you," I said as a warm tear flowed down my face. Healing—the healing journey—had begun. I knew that what was in store for us would not be easy, but together with God, I knew we could face anything put in front of us. Let the healing begin!

Our Miracle Day

I watched in amazement as each day Luke continued to heal and began to walk more and more. He never gave up and continued to push himself to become stable on his new leg. As he became more mobile, I became the opposite. My due date was approaching, and I had gained a hefty amount of weight, so every movement was beginning to be difficult for me. If one more person asked me if I was having twins, I was going to scream. *Don't people know that it is rude to say that to a pregnant woman?* I thought to myself.

I finished the school year with my kindergarteners. The end of the year was a struggle. It was difficult to bend down and tie their shoes and lower myself down to talk to them. I spent the first few weeks of summer lounging in the pool. I would lay my head on one air mattress and my feet on another and let my baby belly hang down in the cool water. It was one of the few ways that I could relax and feel some relief from the heat and pressure all over my body. I enjoyed having the time off with Luke and simply being together. Just being in the same room even if we were doing separate things made me feel close to him.

One hot July afternoon, just five days before my due date, I decided I wanted to get outside and get moving. I reached for my shoes and tried to squeeze my feet into them. The swelling had increased in the previous days, and now my feet were almost unrecognizable. *Will I ever look normal again? Every part of my body is big and bloated, I don't even recognize myself!* I thought. I had long ago stopped looking at the scale and had come to the realization that for the time being I was not going to be my normal size, or even close. I walked out of our bedroom and down the hall. Luke was where I though he would be, on the recliner reading the newspaper.

"Hey, I am going for a walk, maybe go to Target. Do you need anything?" I said as I ran my hands through Luke's baby-soft, newly grown hair.

"No, I am okay. Have fun," Luke said with a smile.

As I walked out the door, I felt confident in the fact that Luke was now able to take care of himself when I was not there. He was getting around very well on his new "leg." The cover was not yet on it, and I did notice a few people stare when we went out in public. It didn't seem to bother Luke too much. I thought back to an incident a few days previous.

I watched through the window as Luke was hosing our lawn. He stood with crutches under his arm, and he was not wearing his leg. I could see the neighbor kids riding their bikes around the neighborhood. Three of them stopped in front of our house, curiosity on their young faces. *What is Luke going to do if they say something? I hope they don't say something rude to him.* I thought.

"Did you break you leg?" I heard a young boy's voice call out.

I couldn't help but laugh. It was obvious to anyone looking that that part of Luke's leg was missing, but I thought it was cute how he asked that.

"No, it was cut off," Luke replied.

Their eyes grew wide, and before they could ask why, Luke continued.

"I had cancer, and they had to cut it off."

"Oh, sorry, man," I heard one of them say, as they hopped on their bikes and rode away. I appreciated that Luke was so calm and patient with them. Children aren't afraid to ask what is on their minds, which can sometimes be refreshing in a world of people afraid to say what they are really thinking.

I set out on my walk. I felt sweat already beginning to bead and form all over my body. The sun shone its powerful rays on me. I was very anxious for my sweet baby boy to come out. I had heard that taking walks and doing lunges can help put you into labor. *It can't hurt!* I thought as I put my right foot far in front of me and I lowered myself slowly toward the ground. It was a difficult task to get op from so low to the ground. I did this several times. *I sure hope it works; I want to meet Hayden as soon as I can!*

I continued my short journey to Target. I entered the store enjoying the cool air that refreshed my flushed body. I walked through aisle after aisle. I was not looking for anything in particular; I just wanted to keep moving. I looked at my watch. Thirty minutes had passed since I entered the store. *I guess that is good enough,* I thought as I headed for the exit. Once outside, the sun instantly made me sweat again. I swept back my blond hair out of my eyes; I had recently had it cut to my shoulders. Since I wasn't feeling good about how I looked, having my hair done helped a little.

On the way back to my house, I did a few more lunges in hopes that it would help start my labor. I returned home and decided my body needed a rest. The evening wore on in typical fashion. Around 10:00 p.m., I began to feel intense pains in my uterus.

"Baby," I said excitedly. "I think I am having contractions."

"Let's wait and see," Luke said calmly. He was used to me thinking that every day was the day that I was going into labor, so he didn't seem to take me very seriously.

I went to our bedroom and lay down to rest. I rested my hand on my stomach.

"Are you ready to meet your mommy and daddy?" I whispered.

Luke sat on the bed next to me. He had a piece of paper in his hand.

"Here comes another one," I said. As each contraction came, Luke would write down what time I had it. He continued by my side doing this for hours. The contractions were now coming quicker and harder.

"I think it is time to go now," I said. I looked at the bright-red numbers on my clock. It read 2:14 a.m. Of course, this would be the time of night Hayden would choose to begin the labor. I rushed around the room to finish gathering things for my overnight bag. I bent over in pain and had to take a break. The pain paused and I continued to get ready. I made my way to the truck and thought about how one of my prayers had already been answered. I thought back to a few months prior, right after Luke's surgery.

"Luke, how do you think we are going to get to the hospital when Hayden comes?" I asked.

"I don't know. Hopefully, I will be able to drive by then," Luke replied.

About a month and a half after Luke's surgery, I came home to Luke waiting to tell me something.

"I drove today, just around the block, but I can do it!" Luke said to me.

"Good job. I am so proud of you," I replied.

"Do you want me to take you for a drive?"

"Yes, that would be fun!" I said as we walked toward the garage.

I stepped up slowly into the truck, carefully trying to keep my balance. I watched as Luke sat down in the truck. He placed his left foot on the brake and his right prosthesis on the gas. We reversed out of the driveway and began down the street.

"Wow, you are doing great. Is it hard driving with both feet?" I asked as Luke drove us around a corner.

"Ya, it's hard because I can't feel the gas pedal with my foot. I feel the pressure at the end of my leg."

We continued down the street and around the block. The truck jerked slightly as we came to a stop sign. Luke looked at me. "It is still a little hard to brake."

"It's okay. You will get better with practice," I said.

We returned to our street and pulled into the garage. Once again, I admired my husband. Most people in his circumstance would never be able to drive and also be so positive.

As I stepped up into the truck this night, I was excited that Luke had taught himself how to drive again and would be able to drive me to the hospital. I checked the backseat to make sure the car seat was there. We had put it there a few nights before so that we wouldn't forget it in the rush to the hospital. Luke sat beside me and got ready to drive.

"Aren't you excited?" I asked in full anticipation of seeing my baby boy for the first time.

"Yes," Luke replied as he yawned. He had a different way of showing emotions, and I knew he was excited but also tired. As we passed the street lights, I felt my anticipation growing. My stomach felt butterflies and I felt as though I was in a beautiful dream.

"Owwww," I wailed as another contraction began. *So much for my beautiful dream,* I thought as I closed my eyes and tried to breathe. We made it to the hospital in seven minutes and pulled into the dark parking lot lit by only a few streetlights.

"Do you think we need to bring in all of our stuff now?" I asked.

"No, let's make sure you really are in labor," Luke said, knowing that sometimes women come into the hospital but are sent home due to false labor.

Luke and I instinctively intertwined our fingers together and walked into the hospital. This was another moment that I had dreamed of my whole life. I savored Luke's touch and felt the warmth of his hand in contrast to the cool night air. We walked to the front desk.

"How can I help you?" the receptionist asked.

"I am having contractions about two minutes apart, and I think I am going into labor," I replied.

"All right, I need your health number," she said.

I fished through my purse and quickly found my insurance card. I handed it to the receptionist.

She typed in my number onto the computer and looked at the screen. Soon a nurse came up to us.

"Right this way, please," she said as she led us down a long hallway and into a small room. I knew the area we were in was the holding area, the place where they were going to check to see if I was really in labor.

Luke found the closest chair and sat down. I knew he was exhausted and his leg was bothering him.

"Please put on this gown and a nurse will come in to check on you in just a minute," I was told as I was handed a pale-blue gown. I was soon dressed and sitting on the bed.

"Luke, Luke, aren't you excited?" I asked emotionally.

"Yes, baby," Luke said. I saw he was struggling to keep his eyes open.

I had never felt this much excitement in my life. The anticipation was building and I couldn't wait to hold my sweet Hayden in my arms. I looked around the tiny room and remembered the day Luke and I had attempted to take a tour of the birthing center.

Just two weeks after Luke's amputation, we were scheduled to take a birthing class in the hospital. He was not feeling up to going, so my mom accompanied me instead. During the second class, Luke felt well enough to go.

We pulled into the hospital and parked in the handicapped parking. Luke maneuvered his way out of the car and onto the sidewalk using his crutches. We walked to the classroom where we found some chairs at the end of a row. As I was pulling a chair for Luke to rest his leg on, people would glance our way but would try not to be obvious about it. *They are trying to figure out what happened to Luke. Whatever, I don't care what they think!*

We sat on the chairs and listened as the instructor talked on and on about birth plans, epidurals, blah, blah, blah. The last few minutes of class were always dedicated to relaxation breathing. The lights were dimmed and we made our way to the floor. My sweet husband, in all his pain, sat behind me. I felt his strong hands begin to massage my back. With all his loving care and tenderness, he continued to do this as the music played.

"I love you," he whispered softly in my ear. The warmth of his breath gave me goose bumps. I felt a wide smile come across my face. *What other husband would do this? Here he is with just his cast, and he came to support me. Most people would probably not even get out of bed. I really am blessed to have Luke!*

Luke came with me one other time. This time, class was to be held inside the birthing center for a tour. We met inside with all the other couples. When everyone had arrived, we began the tour. We took up the rear of the group. Luke was on his crutches. I glanced over at him and saw beads of sweat forming on his forehead. *Oh no, he is sweating. He isn't going to last much longer. I know how he hates to sweat in front of people.*

"I'm going to the car," Luke said as he wiped away sweat from his face.

"All right." I continued on with the group. My heart felt deflated. I knew there were things that were difficult for him, and due to the circumstance, I would have to do some things without him.

I followed the group into a room for new mothers. The instructor was talking but I couldn't hear her words. I looked around the room. Everywhere I looked there were couples. I was the only one alone. *They have no idea how lucky they are just to have their spouses standing next to them.* Suddenly, I had absolutely no interest in hearing about the amenities that the room had to offer. I felt hot tears forming in my eyes. I wanted to be far away from those people. I wanted to be with my husband. I quietly slipped out the door. Trying to hold back my tears, I walked down the hallway and into the parking lot where Luke was sitting in the car. I sat down beside him; and before he could say anything, I said I love you and kissed his lips.

Now, it was the day I was in labor, and I felt blessed to have Luke sitting beside me. Soon a doctor came in and checked on me.

"It looks like you are not quite dilated enough to be admitted. You have a choice; you can either take a walk around the hospital or sit in the whirlpool."

In my mind, there was no hesitating which one I wanted to do. "I would love the whirlpool," I replied instantly.

Luke and I were soon directed to the room with the whirlpool where I was soon basking in a pool of warm water. The jets were directed at my back and eased some of my contraction pains. "I think the water is helping my pain," I said as I leaned back and closed my eyes. I remained in the water for about thirty minutes. The whole time I had been chattering excitedly about Hayden, and Luke had been sitting in the corner in a chair trying to stay awake. I was finally admitted to a room. I had just called my mom, and she came just as we were getting situated in the room.

"I am so excited," she said, and I could see it all over her face. I filled out a million papers, and my pain intensified.

"Are you ready for your epidural?" a nurse asked. I remembered seeing Luke's epidural and thought about how much it had hurt while they put it. I was a bit nervous but ready for some relief from the ever-intensifying pain.

"Yes," I said.

The room cleared out except for Luke. I was directed to sit at the end of the bed. Within a few moments, the epidural was in.

I began to feel warmth spreading throughout my entire body. I knew that the epidural was working, and my relief was beginning. The day progressed without my contractions speeding up. My mother-in-law and my sister-in-law Jessica had arrived during the day as well. Finally, after waiting all day, the time had come for me to push. *I hope this happens quickly. I am ready to hold my baby!* I thought for the millionth time. The pushing began as well as the pain intensity. I noticed that the pain was increasing by the second.

"Is the epidural working?" I said through pain.

"Actually, we had to turn it off. We need to get your baby out now," a nurse replied.

Tears were now rolling down my face, and I was struggling to breathe. My body felt like it was on fire, as if hot flames burned me from the inside. I continued to be instructed to push. Each push lessened my body strength and multiplied my desire to see my baby. I was struggling to breathe and an oxygen mask was placed over my mouth. Luke was at my side, balancing himself on crutches and feeding me ice chips. After a long, difficult push, I looked at him, and tears were running down his face.

"It's so hard to see her in so much pain," I heard him say to my mom. I thought about how interesting it was that our usual roles were now reversed.

Push after push, my body struggled to find energy to continue. Finally, two hours after the pushing began, it was worth every second of the pain. I struggled to push as hard as I could when suddenly a slippery body was placed on top of me. Tears of joy and exhaustion flowed freely down my face.

Luke and I looked at our new baby, our Hayden. A high-pitched cry filled the air, and I had never known such beauty in a cry. Hayden's tiny face looked at mine. His eyes were wide and intent. Luke and I looked at Hayden and then at each other. We kissed softly as I held Hayden in my arms. I felt as if I was in a dream. Luke and Hayden were the only people I could see. The pain was gone from my body, and in that instant, I felt that I was the most blessed woman in the world. Hayden was a miracle from God sent to us when we needed him most. Hayden's tiny fingers wrapped around mine, and I knew that God had given me more than I had ever dreamed or imagined. I stared at Hayden's tiny body and knew that he now depended on Luke and I for his every need. In that precious moment, I realized that I, like Hayden, needed to depend on God for everything. And that everything meant whatever the future might have in store.

Celebrating Our Year

❧❦❧

*C*rash went the cascading waves along the shore. The brisk morning air felt cool and refreshing on my skin. I closed my eyes and let the warmth of the sun transcend upon my body and make its ways deep into the depths of my soul. After all that Luke and I had been through, I felt peace. Not the kind of peace you feel when you have a good day but a peace that goes much deeper. A peace that cannot be explained or understood. God has given it as a miraculous gift.

Thank you, Jesus. Thank you for all you have gotten Luke and I through. You know what you are doing, and I will continue to trust you daily with our future, I whispered softly.

I opened my eyes to see that Luke had joined me on the balcony at our condo. We were at the beach to celebrate our one-year anniversary. It was hard to believe that one year had passed already. So much had happened so quickly.

"You're up early." Luke leaned over to kiss my lips.

"I couldn't sleep. It is so beautiful here," I said as I gazed once again at the vast blue ocean before us.

"I know," Luke replied as he sat down beside me.

"Do you think Hayden is okay?" I asked, thinking of my six-week-old baby. This was the first time we had left him overnight, and I was a little nervous about that.

"I am sure he is fine."

"I miss him," I said. Images of Hayden's precious face filled my mind. As much as I missed him, I was happy to get away and spend time with Luke.

"Me too," Luke said.

Though Hayden had only been with us for six weeks, it was hard to imagine life without him. His cries constantly woke me from my much-needed sleep and his never-ending desire to eat kept me constantly exhausted, but it was the greatest time I had ever known in my life. Luke and I could spend hours staring at Hayden's tiny little features. He already resembled his daddy. He had the same distinct indent in his chin as well as the same face shape. His fingers and toes were so tiny and precious. He was God's amazing gift to us when we needed it the most. He had also been a great source of comfort to me the previous week.

Luke had been getting around the house fairly well with his prosthetic leg for about a month. At night, instead of taking all the time to put his leg on, he would use crutches to get where he needed to go. One night, Luke got up and began crutching toward the bathroom. Suddenly, his crutches slipped as he got to the linoleum, and he began to descend toward the floor. I looked up in time to see him falling. His head came close to hitting my dresser, and he fell and landed directly on the end of his amputated leg. I ran to him and could see the immense pain already overtaking his face. He began to moan.

"Baby, are you okay?" I said intently.

"*Ah*," Luke cried.

Hot tears began to flow down my face. *This cannot be happening. Luke does not deserve this. What should I do?* My mind was racing and trying to decide what to do for my husband.

Luke's moaning became more intense and was beginning to be accompanied by crying.

"Go check on Hayden," Luke said between groans.

"He's fine. I need to make sure you are okay," I said.

"Please, please just go check on Hayden," Luke said. I knew that Luke wanted to be alone in his pain. I quickly but reluctantly left the room and went to Hayden's room just across the hall. I scooped up my tiny baby in my arms and buried my face in his chest. I could hear Luke's muffled cries, and I desperately wanted to make the pain stop. I wanted to take the pain and suffocate its very being. I lifted my face and looked at Hayden. His eyes were staring at me intently. I felt a warm tear drip off my face and onto his. I quickly wiped it off.

"Daddy will be okay," I said as I rocked him back and forth. "Don't worry, baby boy, Daddy will be okay." I realized that the words were meant to comfort myself. I was thankful that Hayden was not older and able to understand the cries of his daddy. *This can't be real. I feel like I am in a nightmare. Who else has to go through this agony? Who can understand this pain?*

I do, my child. I once again hear God's voice speak to me. Yes, God did understand. No earthly person may understand, but God did understand my pain and was holding my hand every moment.

I continued to rock Hayden and let my tears descend down my face, then I picked him up and walked toward our bedroom. I stopped at the door and listened intently. Luke's cries had now subsided, and I decided it was safe to enter. Luke was lying on the bed with his face scrunched up in pain. He was rubbing his leg slowly.

"Hey, are you okay now?" I asked.

"No. I landed right on the end of my leg, right where it is healing."

"I am so sorry," I said as I sat down beside him on the bed.

"It could have been worse," Luke said. "I just about hit my head on your dresser. I could have had a concussion *and* a hurt leg."

"I am really glad that you didn't hit your head," I replied thankfully.

The sounds of the waves brought me back to the present, and I smiled at my husband. I was never happier to be his wife. We had been through so much in just one year. Our year contained more difficult things than most people go through in a lifetime.

"Happy anniversary, baby," Luke said as he reached over to embrace me in a hug.

"Happy anniversary to you too," I said with a smile.

"You know how people say that the first year of marriage is the hardest?" I said.

"Ya."

"Well, what in the world do they have to complain about?" I said with a smile.

"I know," Luke replied. "Let's see, if we didn't have cancer, chemo and amputation, and the challenges of a new baby, what would be difficult?"

"I have no idea!" I replied. I really and truly didn't understand what would be so hard about the first year of marriage without the trials we had been faced with. My mind could not imagine what our first year of marriage would have been like without cancer.

"Do you realize that in our marriage, we have spent more nights in hospitals together than hotels? I think we stayed in the hospital fifteen nights and in hotels eight nights," Luke said.

"Wow, well how about we work on changing that?" I replied.

"If we went through this much in one year, what do you think will we endure next year? It kind of makes me scared for the future," I said.

"Michelle," Luke gently placed his hand on my face. "You cannot spend your life worrying about the future. I could die in a car accident, or you could, or we could live until we are old and gray, but that is out of our control. Only God knows our future. He will take care of us." Luke's deep-brown eyes stared intently at me, as if he were looking directly into my soul. There was no one on earth who knew me better. No one who knew every little detail of my life and loved me in spite of it all. No one who could read my mind with just a glance on my face. No one I would rather be there for in the worst times we had ever imagined.

"I have something for you," Luke said as he got up from his chair and walked into our room.

I wonder what it could be. I'm not really expecting anything, I thought excitedly. I loved surprises.

Luke soon returned with a card that I could tell he had made at home on the computer. On the front there was a picture of a beautiful ocean and underneath it was written "Lincoln City Condo." I laughed aloud.

"I like the picture. Looks just like where we are!"

"I thought you would like that," Luke replied.

I looked down and began reading the card.

Michelle,

This first year of marriage has been the hardest year of my life, but it has also been the best year of my life. Only God, you, my unbelievably loving wife, and the birth of our son has gotten me through. I can't believe how supportive you have been throughout everything. Most women would have given up and left. But you stood by me and even stayed in the hospital with me when you were very pregnant. You are such a trooper, willing to work this year even though you have a newborn that you would like to stay with.

I am sorry that I can't help more, but things will only get better. I promise. We are not the same couple that got married a year ago. We are much more mature and closer. We have truly become one flesh. I am the luckiest man in the world and thank the LORD every day for answering my prayers to have a wife like you.

Your strength, devoutness, and faith have been a testimony in itself to thousands of lives, many of whom we do not even know.

I look forward to many more laughs, cries, adventures, trials and all the good and bad times we are going to have with each other and our family. I would not choose to go through this with any other person ever created. A day in the hospital getting chemotherapy is better than a day anywhere without you. I love you more than I love myself, and I know that you feel the same way.

Thank you, Jesus, for the best, most magical year of my life, with many more to come.

Love,
Luke

I wiped the tears from my eyes and stared at my husband of one year. "Thank you, that was so sweet," I said.

"There is more," Luke said.

"What else could there be, baby? That was more than enough."

Luke handed me a small white box. I opened it quickly as I anticipated the contents. Inside was a thin, shiny, silver bracelet with two tiny diamonds embedded at half-inch intervals. I picked it up and watched the sun sparkle on the diamonds.

"Wow, thank you. It is beautiful," I said as I began to put it on.

"You deserve it," Luke said.

"Well, you told me not to get you much, so I made you something. Let me go get it," I said and walked inside the condo. I grabbed Luke's present out of my bag and returned to the balcony.

"Okay, I have to explain what it is." I held out a two-inch white notebook for Luke to see. On the cover, written were the words "Our Marriage," and underneath was a picture of Luke and I on our wedding day. We were facing each other and saying our vows.

"In this book, I have written what happened to us every month of our marriage. I thought it would be nice to look back someday and remember all the things that we have been through and all the ways that God has taken care of us. I am planning to add to it every year. I hope you like it," I said as I handed Luke the notebook.

Luke silently opened the book and began reading.

August 22, 2004

My Dearest Husband,

One year has passed since the day we said "I do." How quickly the time has flown, but how long I have felt we have been together. So many, many things have changed, yet our love has remained strong. Our love has grown stronger this past year than most people's have in a lifetime. This, without a doubt, has been the most life-changing year I have ever had, and I will never forget it. There are so many memories, good as well as bad.

August 2003

This month was a joyous month; I will never forget the feeling as I was walking down the aisle to you. I could see no one else but you. I loved worshiping God with you at my side. Our first act as man and wife was communion. I was so in awe of God and the way he had blessed me with you that I was overwhelmed with tears and emotions. We prayed together and it was a great moment. That night, we committed our lives to each other in front of all our family and friends. Little did we know what lay ahead for us in the months to come.

September 2003

I was blessed with a new teaching job and was thrown into a whirlwind of activities as soon as I retuned from the honeymoon. You were very supportive, and I really appreciated the way you came to my classroom and helped me set up. You were very cute helping me make charts! We experienced a Ducks game, and we soon realized that football games are not for me! What a great month!

October 2003

Another month of happiness! I remember thinking this is our season for joy; we need to remember this when it is not such a good season. We had fun dressing up as mail carriers for Halloween and helping at our church. The leaves changed colors and you loved the crisp, cool air.

November 2003

This month was an exciting month as we discovered the biggest change in our marriage: we were pregnant! (How did that happen?) You stared at me in disbelief and shock as I took the pregnancy test! You were trying to watch a Ducks game as I was trying to take the test. We couldn't tell if there were two lines or one, so we bought another test; and it was right, we were expecting! Neither of us slept that first night. We were too excited thinking about our new child.

December 2003

I enjoyed our first Christmas together, though I will never forget getting excited about the present that turned out to be windshield wipers! You did a great job with the presents and surprised me with a diamond necklace representing our past, present, and future. We had a beautiful Christmas tree and you put up lights on the outside of the house. You celebrated your twenty-sixth birthday, and we had a quiet New Year's Eve watching a Winterhawks game and coming home and playing the Newlywed Game with Ben and Misty. What a great month!

January 2004

January started off exciting as we got to hear our baby's heartbeat for the first time. What an amazing sound. Things suddenly turned for the worst. You had your biopsy, and on January 23, we heard the devastating results that you had cancer. I remember listening on the phone with you as the doctor explained about it. We held each other and cried and cried. I never felt closer to anyone than you at that moment. Our honeymoon period was over, but we would brave what was to come together. I said in sickness and in health, and I meant it. I was so scared of what lay ahead. You were my strong rock. You kept a positive attitude and helped me fight the anger I was feeling inside. Thank you for being so strong.

February 2004

On February 4th, we found out we were having a boy! I will never forget the look on your face as the news came that we were, for sure, having a boy. It was so exciting to watch our child move around for the first time. We decided on the name Hayden Luke Bader. February was also the month you began chemotherapy. You started getting weaker and losing your hair. I think it was then that the reality of the situation hit me a little more. Like I told you, it was not that I didn't like how you looked without hair; I just didn't like you looking sick.

March 2004

This month started well with a surprise twenty-fifth birthday party for me. I remember that you were not feeling well and that made me sad. You were such a good sport to be there even if you weren't feeling well. The next weekend was not so much fun as it was spent in the hospital. You had your first five-day chemotherapy stay. The nurses were so impressed by your positive attitude, as was I. You impressed me with the way you continued to pray and read your Bible and not be angry. I was angrier than you, and you were the one being pumped with poison for five days straight. I spent my birthday in the hospital, and we ordered Dominos Pizza. We made the best of the situation, thanks to you.

April 2004

In April, you surprised me by saying we could go to Las Vegas for spring break! We had a great time despite the pain in your ankle and my ever-growing belly. We walked through just about all the casinos and wasted our time on driving to Hoover Dam. We lay by the pool, relaxed, and tried to forget the reality that we had waiting for us when we got back home. We had to make the decision of amputation. After weeks of prayer and tears, we decided it would be the best option.

May 2004

May 7th was the most difficult day of our lives. We went to the hospital and were supported by twenty of our closest friends and family as we waited for your surgery. I went back to the preop room, and it took everything in me to hold back my tears. As they wheeled you away to surgery, I felt as if the wind had been knocked out of me. I went to the bathroom and prayed and cried. My heart had never ached so badly for anyone or anything. It was a very long day waiting for you to come out of surgery. I was so proud of you the moment I saw you. You had a smile on your face! Despite everything you had been through, you were smiling! God gave you more strength than I thought was ever possible. As you well remember, that was a terrible night. You were in so much pain and there was nothing I could do. I prayed and cried, cried and prayed. Somehow, the LORD got you through that painful night. We went home, and you began the road to recovery.

June 2004

June was a month that things began to look up; we were excited that you would no longer be doing chemotherapy. It made me nervous knowing that the chemo didn't kill the cancer that was removed, but I learned to trust God that he had it under control. Your hair began to grow back and you began walking on your prosthetic leg! I was so proud of you. I began having contractions and wondered if Hayden might come early.

July 2004

July 7 was by far the best day in our whole marriage. Hayden Luke Bader was born at 5:04

p.m. on that day. The labor was very painful, and you were by my side through the whole thing despite your own pain. The moment they placed Hayden in my arms, it was worth all the pain. I couldn't believe our little miracle was here. God knew that we needed Hayden in our lives at that very moment. He is part of you and part of me. That is truly amazing!

August 2004

Here we are, a year after our marriage began. This month has been a great month. I love when we bring Hayden into our bed and talk to him and watch him coo and smile. He is what has been making us so happy. You are taking me on an amazing overnight trip to the beach. It will be so romantic sitting in our Jacuzzi tub overlooking the ocean. Thank you for the wonderful trip.

It has been a year full of changes. I am glad that God has given me the privilege of being your wife and being by your side for every moment. I wouldn't change it for anything. I pray that this coming year brings a lot more happy times, and we can look back in another year and see how God has blessed us so much in spite of all the pain. I love you, my wonderful, strong husband. I am glad I am your wife now and forever. I love you!

Love always,
Michelle

I continued to observe Luke as he closed the notebook. Tears had begun to fall when he began reading the first page. He looked over at me, reached for my hand, and smiled through his tears.

"Thank you, baby," Luke said. I knew my words had reflected what he was also feeling. We both stood up and embraced in a warm hug. His arms wrapped around me and once again made me feel safe. I looked up at him and our eyes met. His tears spilled onto mine and mixed together. I never felt such peace and happiness. God had helped us survive our first year of marriage, and not just any first year, but a year with difficulty around every corner.

I lay my head on Luke's chest and stared out at the deep, blue ocean. *It seems to go on forever, like my love for Luke. If we can make it through a first year like ours, then we can make it through anything.* We were proof that marriage can survive despite the circumstances. We defied the odds, and God helped us prevail. Our marriage felt stronger and sturdier than marriages that had been together twenty times longer. Our vows were not words said without a backing promise. We understood what they meant and lived them every day. I closed my eyes as I leaned on Luke.

Thank you, Jesus. Thank you for this past year. Yes, it was the most difficult, intense year of my life, but also the best. You showed us how to love each other in the most difficult of circumstances. I want others to see you through us and realize that if you could get us through this, you can get them through anything they are going through. Please use our experiences to help other people. Thank you for showing me how to be a wife of character.

I opened my eyes and stared up at my husband, the most amazing man in the world.

"I love you," I said.

"I love you too," Luke replied.

I closed my eyes again and whispered a prayer of thanks to Jesus. *Thank you for showing me how to love for better or for worse, in sickness and in health.*

I listened to the sound of Luke's heartbeat and realized that despite the trials of the past year, I had been blessed beyond anything I had ever dreamed or imagined.

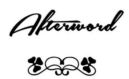

Afterword

*W*e are now approaching nine years since Luke's amputation! We are getting close to the big milestone of ten years cancer-free! We now have three kids. Hayden is eight, Hayley is six, and Payton is four. There have been many struggles, cancer scares, and difficult times, but through it all God remains faithful and has brought us through each valley. We have also had many amazing times as well. Luke gets to be a full-time stay-at-home dad while I continue to run a business from home. Our kids are active, vibrant, and keep each day interesting. We love doing anything and everything as a family. One of our favorite things to do is spend time at "Lake Bader," which is really just our family pool.

We are involved with an amazing church and are surrounded by supportive people who have and will help us in any way possible. Luke still struggles with phantom pain and has many sleepless nights. I do not understand why this still has to happen, but I trust God and am praying for a miracle, that one day the pains will subside. Despite his pain, Luke remains positive and knows that though we still may not understand it; yet, God has a plan for all of this.

We are thankful for the opportunity to share our story and hope it helps countless people know that God is faithful and will help them get through their own journey and struggles. God has taken us by the hand and walked us through each and every trial set in front of us. Through everything, I have learned that God has not forgotten us. He has been with us through everything and will continue to guide and comfort us throughout our lives.

Letters from Friends and Family

My Dear Sweet Luke,

It is hard to put into words how proud I am of you! You have surpassed everyone's expectations of where you would be mentally and physically just a year from your amputation. I knew you were amazing when we got married, but this past year you have amazed me every day with your strength, determination, faith, perseverance, and peace.

I know God has big plans for you, bigger than we can even imagine! He has already used you in so many people's lives that you don't even know about. God chose you. I don't know why he chose you, but he knew that you were strong enough to handle all the things he has put in front of you and come out still serving him. You bring glory to him every day!

You have been such a great example to me in so many ways. When I was angry at God and the world, you showed me how to not have that anger and turn it into peace. You are such a great example to Hayden as well. One day, he will know about the courage of his daddy and hear the story of what happened to you and how you came out praising God! What a wonderful testimony to him and our future children!

I know that sometimes I forget how hard things are for you, and I am truly sorry for that. You never complain and have such a great attitude. I know things are still difficult for you, and I want to help you in every way I can.

My heart has broken with you many times as we have wept, held each other, and cried out to God for answers. Through the pain, we have developed a closeness that cannot be put into words. We have together felt a pain so deep that I believe with all of my heart nothing can separate us. You are my best friend.

You are my hero. You have all the qualities that I want. Hayden and I are by far your biggest fan club.

I am so proud to call you my husband. I honestly think you are the best husband that there is, or has been, or ever will be. You manage to be so wonderful despite all of your pain.

Thank you for loving me and showing me how to draw closer to God through pain. I am forever thankful that God gave me the gift of you!

I love you, my hero.
Michelle

Dear Luke,
It's hard to believe that it's been a year already. It is amazing all the things that you and Michelle went through in the first year and a half of your marriage. We can't believe how God has worked through the whole thing. Your attitude was remarkable through the easy and the tough times. It was so neat to see how God worked through you. We remember when you

guys tithed out of faith and received tenfold of what you gave to go toward your first prosthesis. We are so thrilled that you got to go back to work and move on with your life. You are doing great and are a true inspiration. We both cannot imagine all the scary and awful thoughts that you've had to deal with. You are a real testimony to how God works miracles in our lives.

Love,
Ben & Christie Sims

Dear Luke,

You have been a model of courage, strength, endurance, and patience. You are such an inspiration to those around you.

I am so thankful to God for how he has helped you be so brave through such a very hard season in your life.

We, Mom and Dad, are so proud of you. You are so special.

Philippians 4:13

Love and prayers,
Mom

From Pastor Larry—

On behalf of the pastoral staff at Liberty Bible Church, it is our joy to share of the impact that both Luke and Michelle have had on us. First, we consider ourselves blessed to have you both be a part of this church. There is a sense of pride in knowing that the Bader family attends here.

From the first time we met this couple, we remarked at the spirit and maturity that you possess. The staff talks—sure, we keep things that are confidential—but those character qualities that you two possess have been spoken of on several occasions in the office. We don't have a water cooler where we stand and talk, but we do have a refrigerator that has your picture on it. We've marveled at your courage and faith. You are a true inspiration. The choices that you make as a couple to respond to Luke's health issues are not only wise but motivated by the question "What would God have me to do?" You sought him at every turn. So often, as staff members, we try to be models for the congregation, but you have proven to be models for both the staff and the entire congregation. For this, we commend you. We are blessed as a congregation and are richer because of you.

Jolene McCombs
Secretary
Liberty Bible Church of the Nazarene

Luke,

I know you and I really don't know each other, except for the one or two times that we've been introduced, but I've come to know about you and your story through your lovely wife. And I have to say that knowing a little of what you've been through over the last year and a half, I think you're, well, pretty darn amazing and courageous. It may not feel like it at times, and I'm sure you've had your share of doubts and anger and discouragements along the way, but the fact of the matter is you're still here, and you're still taking it one day at a time. In spite of everything, you've still chosen to be a father, a husband, a son, and a friend…that's everything! You could've chosen differently. You could've let this experience define who you are and tell you how to live your life, but instead you're deciding how your story will be written, and you're letting God take the pen and allow his will to be written across you and your family's life. What a story you will have to share with your son someday when he can comprehend. How he will look up to you and admire the father he has—a father of strength (even when you don't feel like it), courage and commitment to his family and to God. That's a man that he can look up to and aspire to be. Your life choices plant the seeds for generations to come.

Know that you are an encouragement and inspiration to those of us that know your story and that though we don't know each other so well, I am inspired when I think of you and I am reminded to live my life with purpose, courage, and integrity. Know that your example reaches farther than you may ever know, and that God is using you constantly.

Thank you for being the person that you are and for trusting God with your life and setting that example for others.

You, Michelle, and Hayden have been in my prayers since day one, and you will continue to be…always.

Take care, and may God continue to be the guiding influence in your life and in your family.

Kimberly Peterson

Dear Luke,

Oftentimes when I see someone go through trials too hard to describe, I don't know how they do it without Jesus by their side. I've seen you go through a year of trials, and you kept such a sweet spirit and continued to give Jesus praise despite losing a foot. You kept Jesus by your side. I'm so glad you know Jesus and continue to want to give him all the glory. You have inspired me as I've watched from a distance and lifted you to the throne. You have encouraged me as you gave God all the glory for answers to our prayers. What an inspiration to us all. I know God is going to use you abundantly in sharing your trials and "cheering" on someone else who will need your story, prayers, and encouragement in the future. Who knows, it may be your aunt Mary Ann. You are special, Luke. God chose you for a reason. Keep your hand tight to his. I'm anxious to see how he uses you down through the years! Thanks for not giving in to despair when the temptation was definitely there!

Love and prayers,
Aunt Mary Ann

Dear Luke,

Knowing that it is almost a year since you had your surgery, Jerry and I want you to know that you, Michelle, and Hayden are in our thoughts.

You have been an inspiration to us in everything that you have been through. Your faith in God and the strength that you have shown is wonderful.

We so enjoyed Thanksgiving with all of you…made it such a special occasion. It is one of the nicest Thanksgivings that we have had in a long time. Sorry that there was ice on the sidewalk, but thanks to the LORD you weren't hurt bad.

We are so happy that our Michelle married such a super guy and we're glad you are part of our family. You and Michelle have been blessed with such a cute little boy, and he sure looks like his daddy.

Have a great summer, and we hope to be able to come and see everyone this summer. We will always have an extra bedroom available for the three of you, if you ever get a chance to come this way.

Love to all of you,
Phyllis & Jerry

Dear Luke,

Being my brother, I have known you all of your life. Nobody was ever able to get on my nerves, push my buttons, and downright bug me like you did, although I would never have traded you in for something else. I thought it worked out good that I never had to worry about sharing a bedroom.

There were some years when I worried about you, and I would pray for you a lot. Sometimes, I would wake up in the middle of the night and whisper a prayer of safety for you. The LORD still prompts me to pray for you in the middle of the night. I love you very much, and even though we have not been really close the last years and in the same stages in our lives, we share the same parents, and that alone is a bonding experience.

I could not begin to explain how proud I am of you. It's amazing how much you do—from caring for the baby, to taking the garbage out, to going to work all day. I could not begin to understand the physical pain and emotions you go through. What makes you a hero in my eyes, though, is how you have grown closer to the LORD and how you have used this tragedy as a growing experience. I am so thankful that you know the LORD and that you and Michelle are raising your family to be Christ followers. There is great comfort in knowing we will also know each other in heaven! What a great day that will be when we see our Savior!

I will continue to pray and lift you and your family to the LORD. I pray that with each day, the pain will lessen and that you will have wisdom in all your decisions.

You are doing so well with all the "troubles" that have been given to you. Just remember, God won't give you more than he knows you can handle. (I'm guessing that is not always comforting.)

Anyway, in short, I love you, I am always praying for you, and I am proud and amazed at what a man you have turned into.

Love,
Sis

Dear Uncle Luke,

Thanks for always being nice even when you were sick from cancer. Thanks for teaching me how to roller skate. We always had fun jumping on your bed when you lived at Grandma's house!

Love,
Lexi

Dear Uncle,

Thank you so much for loving me all the time. You are a great example to all of us. Thank you for teaching me how to ride a bike. I hope you don't have to go through cancer ever again.

Love,
Your first niece born, jOdEe MaRiE McAlLiStEr

Hello, Luke,

We do not really know each other, but you have always smiled at me and made sure to say hi when you see me! You have touched me in a way that you cannot imagine. You are an inspiration to so many with your faith, honor, and the respect you have for the LORD!

I watched when you were joined with Michelle before God. I came to see Hayden shortly after he was born, and my prayers have been with you through this entire journey. I see (feel) your soul—it is so true and in love with the LORD.

I am not sure you are aware that I suffer from chronic pain, depression, and traumatic stress syndrome. I have had some terrible things happen to me in my short life and after one of those close calls, I found the Lord! He had been knocking for quite a while.

I lost something through being diagnosed with a chronic illness and a mental condition that there is really nothing I can do without taking many doses of medication. Although you cannot physically see my pain, I lost my soul in it. Hearing about what you were going through, I wept to the Lord to hear your prayers for God's will.

I have gained peace by watching you, listening to some of the pain you have gone through and still kept faithful to the Lord. I decided instead of screaming about my pain and depression, I was going to put all my energy into the Lord. If you could, I could, right?

I prayed for you, Michelle, and Hayden when I felt pain. When I prayed for you and family, I felt the Lord take my pain. It was a slight relief; it made me see that the Lord is so great. I was lost, almost ready to give up on him; all I could see is failing, failing God, falling back into old ways. I know God has a bigger plan for me than to suffer day after day.

I want you to know that you are a huge part of why I remain in my walk with the Lord.

Now faith is confidence in what we hope for and assurance about what we do not see. This is what the ancients were commended for. By faith we understand that the universe wsa formed at

God's command, so that what is seen was not made out of what was visable

—Hebrews 11:1–3, NIV

The word of God states that "whatsoever is not of faith is sin" (Romans 14:23b). Romans 12:3b **says,** "God hath dealt to every man the measure of faith." We are then to allow the Holy Spirit to move in our lives so that our faith might grow in him. For faith to grow and for God to honor our faith, there are several principles we must follow in the word of God, since faith alone cannot produce our prayer answers.

Your faith has shined through to my heart…

Tiffany Tremaine

Hello, Mr. Bader,

I just wanted to let you know how impressed I am with how you have handled everything that life has thrown at you in the last year or so. I'm told that the LORD will never give us more than we can handle. He must think that you are a superman. I have come closer to him recently, and I have a long way to go. I struggle with my spirituality daily, but he always seems to give me little reminders to bring me back up. I wish for you continued strength, to become closest to God, and much deserved happiness for your future.

God bless,
Sherry Jones

Luke~

Congratulations on your one-year mark of your surgery! We are excited to see how far you have come from this time last year. We wanted to share with you something you probably didn't know. When you got sick last year, we put you and Michelle and unborn Hayden on our church prayer list, and then we called a couple of other churches in the area and put you guys on theirs, too. We asked a couple of friends to pray also. We were thinking and praying for you often and would update people on how you were doing. As time passed, the people we had told to pray for you had put you on other prayer lists and told their friends to pray for you too. Throughout the year, we have been told about so many people and so many prayer lists that you have been on. The greatest part about this is that so many people have got to hear that the prayers they prayed for you were answered. It has been such an awesome testimony to be able to tell everyone who is often asking about you that you are doing so great. It's so encouraging to know that there is an awesome network of believers who are spread out around the nation who will pray for you and believe that God would heal you. We know that you still have a lot more to go through and still have hard times and hard days. But we are all still praying for you and believing that God has an awesome plan for your life!

We know that it's not exciting to be a cancer survivor when you never wanted to have cancer in the first place. But we are so glad that you are a survivor and that you are here, and that your beautiful son can play and grow up with our daughter!

With his love,
James & Monica Hill

Luke,

I am sure that this past year has been a blur of days and events. Many days were filled with the unknown and probably a lot of different emotions—some not so good days, and some so very beautiful (the birth of your son).

The thing that I find so amazing, Luke, is that you, through it all, have remained constant and steady with your love for God, fully trusting and leaning on him for your strength and for the unknown. Your courage and strength is a real testimony to anyone that knows the storybook fairy tale of you and Michelle and how that story took a really unexpected and nasty turn. And yet, you never became resentful or bitter toward your Father in heaven.

Luke, you have been a real witness to many people that you are not even aware of. And the testimony you and Michelle have is a really amazing thing.

Our prayers are still with you and your little family. We pray that God will continue to use you both to touch the lives of others. It's a beautiful thing when God's children can take a situation that Satan meant for evil and harm and turn and use it for the glory of God. It's like that old saying "using lemons to make lemonade."

We love you both…all three of you. Our thoughts and prayers are with you.

Love,
Sherry Boswell

Luke,

You have made such a difference in each one of our lives, and we continue to learn from you and your experience.

It is so amazing to see how God set the pieces of your life in place just perfectly before your cancer was detected. God gave you a job at the US Postal Service where you received great health insurance and met some wonderful Christian men who were constantly praying for you and encouraging you. You were also reunited with Michelle (an awesome woman of faith) whom you married shortly after. The timing of you both finding such a great church that took you under their wing and then getting pregnant with the little angel, Hayden, (or "little Luke"). As we look back at how God placed the pieces together in your life prior to being diagnosed with cancer, we truly are reminded of God's faithfulness to those who follow him.

From the moment you told Aaron that you had cancer, you have had the most positive attitude. We remember the car ride when Aaron got the call from you. We both said a prayer right away and then Aaron stated, "Luke is such a strong person, he can beat this." Today, Aaron looks back at that day and thinks, "I knew Luke was a strong person, but to see one of my best friends go through such a tough year and a half and come out with a great attitude is remarkable. That guy is even stronger than I had imagined." Along this difficult journey, God has given you so many reasons to live. Hayden is just one of the joys God has given you that show his perfect timing. His birth came at a perfect time to remind you and all of us just how precious life is here on earth, and to give you another reason to fight this cancer. Your son will be so proud of you, Luke, whether it be chemotherapy or radiation. Even after your amputation, your face shined with life every time we were around you. You are a true testament of God's unfailing love. He has used you and molded you into an even better man; one we hope our boys can grow up to model after. Ethan and Kaden have actually already learned so much from you. They both are in awe of your courage and the way you haven't given up along the way. They think you are a superhero. You have taught them to trust in the LORD, to have patience, and the importance of prayer. Thank you for that. God is using you in ways I bet you didn't even know about.

Thank you for every moment of faith you have had. We never once saw your faith in God waver. You trusted in the LORD every step of the way with a smile on your face. Your faith gives us hope. The world needs more people like you. Thank you for your inspiration, your strength, your love, and your smile.

Love,
Aaron, Susanne, Ethan, and Kaden Watzig

Luke,

As I sit down to write this letter to you, I am overwhelmed with emotions and memories of the times we have had together. I will always remember sitting in your living room, hanging out and spending time together in fellowship and in the Word. That group was so important to me and helped me in my walk with the LORD and in balancing my life and ministry. But more than that group, you were an inspiration to me and a true friend. I think for me, our relationship was a godsend.

There was a reason that God brought you into my life, and as I watched you in the past two years, it was evident why. I had never truly understood what it meant to trust in the LORD. I had never personally grasped what true faith in the Almighty God meant. To watch you was a humbling experience because I cannot say for sure that I would have been as strong as you were. You stood there, amidst all that was being thrown at you, and you shined. The light of Christ was never more evident to me in any one person as it was when I would look at you. You have an unbelievable character and a faith that is as solid as the Rock it is built on.

It is amazing to me how strong you were, how you continued to lead your family spiritually, and how you continued to lead those in your small group. You may not think you were leading us, but you were. Each week was a reminder of the faithfulness of God, even when it was difficult to see it with our human eyes. All I could think of was that you were too young to have this happen to you. You had just gotten married, you were having a son; it just was not fair! But those words *never* came out of your mouth. All we heard you say was how you desired for God to use this to impact people. All you spoke of was your faith and trust in the Almighty God whom you knew would pull you through!

I will never forget the voicemail that I got when Melissa and I had gotten the call to go to Nampa. You had no clue what was going on but just responded to the leading of the Holy Spirit. You called me and said how you just knew that you needed to pray for me, and that the LORD had laid me on your heart. As I listened to that message, it blew me away. Your sensitivity to the LORD is incredible, and your care for others regardless of your situation is truly amazing. I will never forget that day.

God has done a miracle work in your life. He did not take everything away and make it perfect, but he truly did use you to make a difference in his kingdom. You may never know how much you mean to Melissa and me and how much I look up to you, but I hope this letter has begun to capture some of how I feel. I am proud to call you friend and blessed to have had you in my life for the time I did. I miss your bright smile and your passion for life. I miss walking in your front door and knowing that you would be there waiting to hear how I was doing.

We are thinking of you guys and praying for you. May God continue to richly bless you and your family. May you be blessed in the same way that you have blessed so many people!

In his grip,
Nathan & Melissa Roskam

Dear Luke,

It is hard to believe that it has already been a year and a half since you started your battle with cancer. It has been absolutely amazing to see what God has done in your life. Some of the really simple things have made such an impact in our lives. It seems like every time we came to your house or went to visit you in the hospital, I noticed your Bible beside your chair or sitting on your bed stand. It has been such a testimony—a true sign—that you were seeking God and calling out to him during a difficult time in your life.

I am sure all of us can think of a time or two in the past when we thought we could handle it all on our own, and now as we look back, we can see how much easier it would have been to call upon God who was there all along just waiting for us to seek him!

These last several weeks, Ben and I have been putting some thought into how God has used your experience to touch our lives...I am sure we could come up with a list that goes on and on, but we felt impressed to share some with you...I know that by now it probably sounds cliché, but Luke, through your experience, we have truly learned to enjoy some of the more simple things in life. We have experienced how thankful we are to have you as a friend, and in that same breath, we have realized how precious life is and that we need to not take it for granted.

Luke, during this past year and a half, I have learned a side of Ben that most will probably never get to experience. I have tried to come up with an adjective that describes Ben, but the best I could come up with was "self-sacrificing." When Ben first learned that you had cancer, Luke, he was *so* concerned. He wanted to be there for you, but he didn't want to talk about the cancer if you didn't want to; but on the other hand, if you wanted to talk, he wanted you to know that you could talk to him. He wanted to help you, but yet if you didn't want help, he didn't want to force himself on you. The one thing, though, that has made a huge impact in my life was when you first told us that you were going to have your leg amputated. After you told Ben, he told me right away, and he looked at me and said, "Why can't it be me?" I immediately turned to him and said, "How can you say that? How can you wish it was you?" I don't mean to say that I am glad it was you and not us, but I felt so angry at Ben for saying that. I didn't understand what Ben was thinking.

It wasn't until a few weeks later that it dawned on me...Ben's love for you, his friend, is so strong, and he is so loyal that he couldn't stand the thought of you being in pain and having to deal with this. If Ben can love you enough to want to take this battle from you, *how much more does God love us to give his one and only son to die on the cross for us?* I know that until

I have children of my own I will not be able to understand a parent's love for their children, but I think I have a renewed sense of how absolutely amazing it was for God to give his son for us.

Luke, you have been a tower of strength throughout this past year and a half. I am sure that there are weak moments, but it has been amazing to me the strength you have had and the positive outlook you have maintained. God is working in your life to touch each of us, Luke!

Your friend,
Misty

Luke,

These past few weeks, I have taken some time to reflect on this past year and the impact you have had on my life. Luke, your diagnosis was a wakeup call for me, as it was the first experience I have had with cancer. It made me take a look at the way I was living my life and highlighted the things that I needed to change. Through your experience, you have shown the peace that God can provide even in the midst of turmoil. I have in my own life dealt with health issues that have caused me to at times feel sorry for myself. Your eagerness to look for ways to help others and impact their lives has shown me that I need to look to God for ways to use my experiences. I know that there have been, and probably will be, times when you are down, but I want you to know that your willingness to look to God for help has left a lasting impact in my life.

Ben

Luke,

As you recover, you're kept in mind with the warmest of thoughts, and you're kept in heart with "special prayers" that God will bless you. You have been an inspiration.

Michelle,

Appreciate your support! May God bless you both.

Love,
Aunt Ellen

Luke,

I hope one day you look back at the past year of your life as one where you can say "Thanks, LORD, for the trials I went through." 2 Corinthians 12:7–10 has been so real to me lately...*Am I strong enough to be weak?* When I have to sit and watch Dave do my housework? When people stare at me when I'm being pushed in the wheelchair? When I'm having constant pain in my legs?

I know, Luke, you are strong enough to become weak, letting Christ be your strength.

I'm sure you and Michelle have had many exciting and happy times the past ten months, watching your precious son, Hayden, grow and learn, and will have many more years to do so.

Praise the LORD for your first anniversary of success with the *big challenges* you have faced and completed.

Love,
Aunt Donna

Luke,

I have been praying for you since the moment I knew that Michelle was growing in my womb. It was amazing to see how God protected Michelle and kept her until both of you were ready to become a family, and to watch as the two of you have started your life together. Even when we found out that you had cancer and that things were going to get pretty tough for both of you, I had no doubt that you were the man that Michelle needed to be her husband and partner. I continue to thank God for you being her husband and our "son."

I admire the way you have kept your good attitude and have relied on God to get you through. It was such a witness of God's grace to see both you and Michelle with a positive attitude when you were in the hospital. Even when you were going through such hard times, you would have a smile. I am so thankful that God decided to give Hayden to you during this time. He is such a blessing to all of us, and I was so thankful for the two of you to have something positive to focus on. I admired your strength when Michelle was in labor. You had just gone through so much yourself, but you wanted to make sure you could be right there with her and for her. The joy on both of your faces when Hayden was born was wonderful to see, and the way both of you have taken the responsibility of parenting is something I am so thankful for. I will keep praying for the three of you as you continue to grow into the family that God wants you to be.

Some of the things that have been an encouragement during this hard time are the way God took care of financial needs for you. It was overwhelming to see how it all fell together and how God really put a burden on Sherry to get things organized. The way people gathered around not just in the financial but the many other ways (such as having your lawn mowed and cared for) was such a blessing to see. God showed his love for you through a lot of friends and family.

The following verses have been ones that have helped me through a lot of life's problems:

For I know the plans that I have for you, declares the Lord, plans for welfare and not for calamity to give you a future, and a hope.

—Jeremiah 29:11

Trust in the Lord with all of your heart, lean not on your own understanding, in all your ways acknowledge Him, and He will make your paths straight.

—Proverbs 3:5–6

Love,
Your other Mom, Karen

Brother Luke,

It is with a great honor and respect that I get to sit here and write to you this letter. I will have a combination of scripture and thought for you as it develops. Hope you enjoy it.

In your life, the story can relate for "What did you do to deserve this?" God, if he wanted, could do even greater to punish you for the sins you committed. The Bible states God tempts no man with evil. If you are tempted, it's not from God! The Bible also states "every good and perfect gift comes down from the father." You can find this for yourself in James chapter one. In this battle, God gives you this word of encouragement: "I will never leave you or forsake you"—you can read this in Hebrews 13:5—and "He takes the ashes of the evil works and out of them he will create beauty." Saul's grandchild was crippled and wounded in the battle, just as you were, waiting upon a move from the LORD. When the time came, he had a choice to make—he could choose to blame all that had happened to him upon God, or he could stand before him and hear what it was that God wanted to do with him. He, as you, made the choice to hear what God wanted to do with him. As you can see by the story, God's choice was to bless him and to restore him. Luke, in order for God to do this, Saul's grandchild had to take a scary course of action. Are you ready for that? Mephibosheth had to face what he thought was his enemy and know that God had his best at heart. Not an easy action for him to make, totally vulnerable; no protection from the *fear* of consequences. One thing is sure about the LORD: He knows what it takes to make us rely fully on him.

Now after Mephibosheth is completely restored, King David ends up in hiding because his son is trying to steal the kingship from him. To shorten the story, David's son's plot is destroyed, and his son dies. After this, King David is being put back in power. It is at this time that Mephibosheth sends his servant out to meet the king.

Sometimes, when we think all is well, we have failed to realize how our enemy will never quit or stop. Let's see what happens next as David returns to Jerusalem himself.

It is not until this moment, a moment like this, that God's work in us is complete. For even when it is more profitable for us personally if we would have taken another route, we still stand for God. With King David being in exile, it would have been a great time to make a move to finish destroying the king, and yet Mephibosheth, as his dad, chose servanthood.

In you, Luke, I see so much, and even more than what I wrote for you of this story.

Luke, I, as Christ, can only say I love you—really love you—my brother. No, I mean *really* love you.

You are more than a brother—you're an inspiration to me and to my family. I know that in Christ, you have so much he wants to do with you.

In closing this, let me say: As much as I see in you, Christ sees even more and more and more. Just let him finish the good work he has started in you, and he will supply all of your needs.

Love always,
Your brother in Christ, RG Paschall

It's hard to put in words how Luke inspires me. My son Phillip left last August to start basic training for the army. We would get letters almost every day telling us how hard it was. Lucky for us, he was given a Bible when he got to basic. I suggested he read 1 Corinthians 10:13. It talks about being tempted and how God will never give us more than we can handle. I believe that goes for all other aspects of our lives. I think sometimes that God has shown Luke the very edge of what anyone could handle. That inspires me. I look at what I and others complain about in our lives and see Luke in the next case at work and tell myself, *What am I thinking?* My little piddly problems are miniscule, and yet Luke keeps rolling along, never voicing his displeasure. That's a real man. I'm very proud of that guy and consider myself lucky to be able to spend time working, talking, and laughing together.

Man…I love you, man. I love you, man.

Dennis "Elwood" Hickox

May the LORD bless Luke, Michelle, Hayden and the whole Bader family.

Luke,

With your cancer and subsequent amputation, you have grappled with physical extremes that most of us have not and yet seem able to retain a positive attitude through it all. I am impressed with your resiliency and pleased that you have been an inspiration to many.

I trust that you will continue to view life through the lens and vantage point of God's wisdom rather than your own. He has brought you through a set of circumstances that I can't understand but am convinced of their value in your life, in the lives of your family and within your sphere of influence. Look daily to what you might learn from your unique position and be the spiritual head of your household as God has called you to be. "I have no greater joy than to see my children walk in the truth" is a reality to me, and now you have become a part of that lineage and a major contributor to one branch of the family tree. Please allow your "limitation" to be a source of strength and your life an encouragement to those around you.

Papa Rommel

Luke,

What a difference a year makes! And who knew so much could happen in that mere year? I wanted to say a few things to you, and I guess this is my best attempt, so bear with me. I know you've heard it many times, but all of us who love Michelle were afraid for her for a while that we would lose her and "prayed our knees off" that God would send someone who would cherish and value her. Never have I ever had such a feeling of peace for her as I did when I met you. You have been a steady and strong anchor for her, which she needed. Through all that has happened, I just kept thinking, *Why God? Why Michelle, when she is finally in a good place? Why Luke, Lord, when he is one of the good ones?* But God just kept saying the same thing over and over, "Watch and learn." So I did, and I have. You have been such a pillar of faith. You know from whom your strength comes from, and those who see you do also. You cared for Michelle and made sure she had what she needed during the pregnancy. Your determination and commitment to getting better was so inspiring. You taught me a lesson in faithfulness in tithe which I needed to remember. But the one thing I learned from my watching you the last year was God can't fill us unless we empty ourselves, and we aren't empty if we are filled with self-pity.

I don't think God minds whys, but he prefers hows. Why now for Michelle? Because she is finally in a good place. Why Luke? Because he is one of the good ones. He knew you could do this, Luke, and he knew how it would touch all of us around you for his glory. Thank you. Thank you for your strength, your conviction, your willingness to endure this and let us watch and differently learn.

All my prayers,
Di Adra Rose

Luke,

You have been an inspiration to us all, even when you are not meaning to. Your actions through times of trial set the bar for all of us to follow. Tragedy hits us all at some point in our lives, and when it is my turn, I will remember your example. Thank you for your faith in God and your strength.

Kevin Rose